DATE DUE

OCT1 9 1994	

GAYLORD

PRINTED IN U.S.A.

NAMELESS
DISEASES

NAMELESS
DISEASES

▲▲▲

Terra Ziporyn

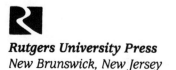

Rutgers University Press
New Brunswick, New Jersey

Copyright © 1992 by Terra Ziporyn
All rights reserved
Manufactured in the United States of America

Library of Congress Cataloging-in-Publication Data

Ziporyn, Terra Diane, 1958–
    Nameless diseases / by Terra Ziporyn.
        p.   cm.
    Includes bibliographical references and index.
    ISBN 0-8135-1800-8
    1. Chronic diseases.   2. Nosology.   3. Medical misconceptions.
    I. Title.
    RC108.Z56   1992
    616—dc20   91-36660
                                                            CIP

British Cataloging-in-Publication information available

To Lester Snow King

CONTENTS

▲

ACKNOWLEDGMENTS

Many volunteer readers and critics helped to transform this book from a vague glimmer that came to me years ago as I flew from one medical conference to another. I owe particular gratitude to the thoughtful and sometimes painfully honest suggestions of Jerry Weinberg, Cheryl Plum, Elizabeth Knoll, Dr. Warren Newton, Dr. Marvin Ziporyn, and both of my brothers, Brook and Evan Ziporyn. I also want to thank Bruce Lewenstein, who allowed me to present some of these ideas to a critical audience at Cornell University. Long-overdue thanks also go to the American Association for the Advancement of Science and the Searle Family Fund, whose Mass Media Science Fellowship and Searle Fellowship, respectively, helped provide the dual perspective—medical writing and medical history—on which this book rests.

Donna Morgan and Jeffrey Hansen of the Myalgic Encephalomyelitis Association, Mary Lou Ballweg of the Endometriosis Association, Kathy Hunter of the International Rett Syndrome Association, Orvalene Prewitt of the National Chronic Fatigue Syndrome Association, Rosemary Bowler of the Orton Dyslexia Society, and Dr. Channi Kumar of the Marcé Society all contributed valuable literature about the nameless diseases represented by their organizations. And although I cannot list them by name, I am deeply grateful to all the people suffering from "nameless diseases" who shared their stories with me and without whom I would have been unable to write this book.

Special thanks go to Steve and Selina Collier, who read successive versions of the manuscript with critical and constructive eyes. I will be forever grateful for the rare courage of conviction that kept them believing in the book through its darkest moments. Their devotion was matched only by that of my husband, Jim Snider, who not only read and relentlessly critiqued every word, but grasped the book's significance perhaps even more than I did. Without his faith, encouragement, and practical suggestions, *Nameless Diseases* may never have escaped the confines of my word processor.

NAMELESS
DISEASES

INTRODUCTION

▲

When Experts Disagree

As a medical writer I frequently witness a phenomenon rather foreign to most nonphysicians: the medical meeting. At these scientific forums, generally held at elegant hotels and conference centers, leading researchers from around the world present research findings so recent that they haven't yet hit the medical journals. These meetings provide a treasure trove of information for medical journalists, who meet in the pressroom to discuss the most exciting papers and to interview the speakers. These meetings also, however, present a disturbing conundrum: again and again, the findings of one reputable researcher directly contradict the findings of another equally reputable colleague.

I've been puzzling over these contradictions for many years now. One study says that people with diabetes have an immunity problem; another says that there is no known mechanism for diabetes. One study contends that drugs can cure women of dysmenorrhea (severe menstrual cramps); another says that this condition is "all in the head." One study says that 10 percent of the population suffers from learning disabilities; another says that the figure is only 1 percent.

As I sit through these scientific sessions and listen to these conversations, I keep asking myself "What's the matter here?" The first answer that pops into my head is that some investigators must be doing valid research while others are not. But reviewing the evidence, I find that in most cases this just isn't true: most scientists presenting their data at national and international meetings have conducted legitimate studies, all using proper control groups, statistically significant sample sizes, and logical analyses.

My gut reaction has to have been wrong, then. It seems that results are contradictory, despite valid experiments. I know, of course, that science is full of uncertainty—my studies of medical history have taught me that—but this particular sort of uncertainty seems to me to make a mockery of experimental science. If there is such a thing as objective truth, I reason, then how can several different scientists doing perfectly valid investigations come up with such different results? It seems almost as if everyone is looking at a different universe.

And then one day it hit me: they *are* looking at different universes. Time after time, investigators claim to be researching a specific "disease," but each investigator defines this disease in a slightly different way. Without a standard definition, no study can be compared with any other. One researcher, for example, may have defined chronic fatigue syndrome as including anyone who feels tired most of the time, while her colleague may have restricted it to persistent fatigue coupled with flu symptoms and perhaps even an associated virus. It's no wonder, then, that they get different results. Furthermore, without an agreed-on definition, more sophisticated correlations and predictions become meaningless. If you don't know what chronic fatigue syndrome is, for example, how can you say what happens to people with chronic fatigue syndrome?

I started to realize just how pervasive this definition gap was when I thought back to many other meetings I had covered. Whether the subject was chronic fatigue syndrome, premenstrual syndrome, dyslexia, puerperal psychosis, scoliosis, diabetes, or cancer, I could never get a straight story as to what precisely characterized a given disease. I remember quite vividly, for example, having lunch with several doctors one day in Anaheim's Disneyland Hotel, at a meeting on premenstrual syndrome. The family practitioner next to me was describing one of his patients. "Premenstrual syndrome is a real problem," he said, "and it's time we did something about it. Why, just last week the husband of one of my patients called me up and said his wife was about to get her period and had just hit him over the head with a wine bottle."

Several doctors across the table immediately stopped cutting their chicken kievs.

"That's right," the family practitioner continued. "The poor woman just can't control herself on those days. Last month, in fact, she hit her husband with a flowerpot."

I was madly jotting all this down in my notebook when a gynecologist on my left spoke up. "I don't buy that at all," he said. "In my opinion, premenstrual syndrome is just a line mentally ill people use to excuse their behavior. For God's sake, in England they're literally letting women get away with murder, just for claiming they have premenstrual syndrome."

"Isn't there some way to tell whether or not a woman has this thing, this premenstrual syndrome?" I asked naïvely. Surely there had to be some easy way of telling whether a woman had the disease or was merely faking. "If only we knew," both doctors replied.

This bothered me. I couldn't understand how people could spend year after year studying something that they couldn't even define. But it happens all the time. Several months earlier on the opposite coast, I recalled, I had attended a meeting on dyslexia. Because I was writing for a medical journal, I felt that my first duty to my readers was to characterize this condition, which is better known among psychologists and educators than among practicing physicians. I knew that all people with dyslexia have certain specific difficulties with language, but I wanted to find out what other characteristics distinguished them, since not all people with these language difficulties have dyslexia.

Unfortunately, I couldn't get a straight story. I heard one psychiatrist tell a roomful of scientists and educators: "Kids with dyslexia 'perseverate.' Once they start any activity they stick to it ad nauseam." "Good," I thought, as I noted that children with dyslexia are persistent. But then, less than a half hour later, a clinical psychologist at the same meeting told me that "one common trait in kids with dyslexia is that they can't concentrate on anything. They have what we call an 'attention-deficit disorder.'"

Hearing that, I tore up my notes and started to wonder whether the psychiatrist's "dyslexia" was the same thing as the clinical psychologist's. Was there really such a disease as dyslexia, or was "dyslexia" merely a convenient term to describe a certain kind of behavior—that behavior being merely a symptom of one or more comprehensive diseases? The latter idea might explain the differences between the statements I had heard. Maybe one person had a brain tumor which caused reading disabilities and attention deficits. Maybe another had a birth defect which caused "perseverance and reading disabilities." If so, did these two people have the same *disease*—dyslexia—or did they merely share one *symptom*—language disability?

The need for good definition seemed straightforward enough. So straightforward, in fact, that I couldn't quite believe it accounted for the contradictions and confusion I kept witnessing. Certainly good researchers know to define their terms, don't they? Yes, they usually do. Surely I couldn't be the only one noticing the confusion at these meetings. The researchers themselves must be fully aware that one study does not mesh with the next. Yes, again, they usually are. But, amazingly enough, only rarely do researchers define exactly what they mean by the "disease" under investigation.[1]

It turns out, in fact, that most practicing doctors and scientists, with the exception of a few academic psychiatrists, are able to justify discrepancies without tackling this rather vague, philosophical issue.[2] While some merely accuse colleagues of invalid research, most deal with contradiction by assuming that their colleagues are merely looking at different aspects of the same phenomenon. Once the entire disease is understood, they argue, the contradictory states will be reconciled.

In other words, most doctors and investigators who speak at medical meetings simply assume that they are indeed talking about the same "disease." Philosophers of medicine and some textbook writers may ponder such issues, but in the day-to-day work of practitioners and researchers, they are assumed to be settled. By giving a set of conditions a name, by calling it by the name of one specific disease, everyone feels that there *is* only one thing, and that they are all talking about that very same phenomenon.

When I started to think some more about these assumptions, I realized that you didn't have to go to medical meetings to feel their impact. A headline in the morning paper would scream "New Drug Cures Diabetes," only to be followed the next day by "Doctor Says New Diabetes Drug Has Limited Potential." From what I could tell, the sources for both articles were legitimate, so whom was I to believe? Another page proclaimed "Cancer Treatable with Hormone Injections," while an ad promised "full recovery from cancer with vitamin pills."

And then I thought of the patients themselves. After all, when a patient comes to the doctor with a complaint (a symptom), the doctor's first task is to make a diagnosis—specifically, to fit the symptom or combination of symptoms into a coherent pattern, that is, a disease.

Say John comes in and complains that his stomach aches midmorning almost daily and usually aches again several hours after eating. The doctor does a physical exam, asks a few questions, runs some laboratory tests, and hopes that she finds enough clues: perhaps a "crater" in an X-ray picture and John's acknowledgment that the pain goes away after eating. If the doctor finds enough clues suggesting a consistent pattern, she may make a *diagnosis:* "duodenal ulcer," for example. She may then prescribe a *therapy:* tranquilizers, a modified diet, and antacids, perhaps. She may also give John a *prognosis:* the ulcers will heal in two to six weeks but probably reappear in the next several years. The doctor can determine this diagnosis, therapy, and prognosis—or, as some medical philosophers would put it, she can explain, control, and predict—because, in today's medical books, "duodenal ulcer" is considered a disease and thus has certain associated characteristics.

Now consider another patient, Joe. Although Joe has complaints similar to John's, the doctor finds no evidence suggesting lesions in the duodenum. And so, ruling out duodenal ulcer, the doctor looks for other likely explanations, perhaps food poisoning, a history of food allergies, or infection by a microorganism. But none of these guesses proves correct either. The doctor who cannot fit observations into a known category then has several alternatives:

1 *Blaming the patient.* Here the doctor tells Joe, "It's all in your head" or "You're a hypochondriac" or "If you took better care of yourself, this wouldn't have happened." This sort of response is quite common when there is little scientific evidence available to explain a symptom or condition. Until a few years ago, for example, gynecologists were notorious for smiling condescendingly at women with dysmenorrhea and telling them that their cramps would disappear if only they accepted their femininity. Only when researchers began documenting that many women with severe menstrual pain also had abnormally high levels of prostaglandins did doctors start offering women medicine instead of blaming them.

   As Susan Sontag writes in *Illness as Metaphor,* "Theories that diseases are caused by mental states and can be cured by will power are always an index of how much is not understood about the physical terrain of a disease."[3] Western society tends to blame the victim for suffering if it cannot find anything else to blame. Popular articles, furthermore, constantly emphasize the poor personal habits associated with such baffling medical conditions as cancer, diabetes, heart disease, and alcoholism. Because we don't know the specific causes of these conditions, we promote "healthy" practices as the best way to prevent them; then we assume that anyone who gets sick must have neglected these practices. Of course, poor diet and exercise habits may indeed underlie certain medical conditions, but consider this: a century ago, before scientists had traced infectious diseases to specific microorganisms and had affirmed that sanitation, vaccines, and antitoxins could control them, Americans tended to link typhoid, cholera, and diphtheria—diseases that we now link with infectious microorganisms—with immorality or slovenliness in their victims. Such judgments often continue until scientists discover a specific external cause.

2 *Misdiagnosing the patient.* Joe's doctor doesn't do this maliciously, but simply makes the best guess he can based on his limited evidence. He might tell Joe, for instance, that he has "gastroenteritis," which is a generic term for a variety of conditions that may very well include Joe's. Joe does not know that this guess is at all tentative, however; he thinks his doctor has pegged the problem. And so, Joe goes home, happy (for a while at least) to know what he has and what to do about it. Only later, if the treatments don't work or he grows sicker, will Joe suspect the mistake.

3 *Retesting or referring the patient.* Finding no explanation for Joe's stomach problems, the doctor offers him further testing or refers him to another doctor. Thus, Joe adds to his time and expense, his worry and uncertainty. If the disease causing his stomach problems is never "discovered," he once again faces alternative 1 or 2.

4 *Admitting ignorance.* The doctor tells Joe the truth; that is, "I don't know what disease you have or if you have a disease at all." It is the rare doctor honest enough to admit this, and the rare patient willing to accept it.

From everything I saw, then, diseases that lacked clear definitions led patients to additional suffering and led researchers to all sorts of contradictory conclusions. That the lack of a simple definition could have such far-flung repercussions didn't make sense to me, however.

Why couldn't researchers just define which observable phenomena constitute each known disease, syndrome, or symptom? Why couldn't doctors just fit a patient's characteristics into these definitions? Why should that be so difficult?

Only after long talks with doctors, long nights with medical texts, and long chases through dictionaries did I find my answer. No one knew what it meant to call something a disease in the first place. Even within the medical profession—even in the lexicon of the same doctor—there is no standard usage of terms such as "disease," "illness," "sickness," "syndrome," or "disorder." When I went to a standard medical dictionary, one used by the editors of a major medical journal, and looked up "disease," I found this definition: "a definite morbid process having a characteristic train of symptoms; it may affect the whole body or any of its parts, and its etiology, pathology, and prognosis may be known or unknown."[4]

If diseases were processes made up of "symptoms," the logical next step was to find out what a symptom is. The dictionary entry read: "any subjective evidence of disease or of a patient's condition, i.e., such evidence as perceived by the patient; a change in a patient's condition indicative of some bodily or mental state."[5] Any time a doctor saw a sick patient, so it seemed, the only question to settle was whether the condition was "a definite morbid process" with "characteristic symptoms" or whether there was "subjective evidence of disease."

But as I looked more carefully at those authoritative dictionary entries, I realized that I had run up against the great problem of dictionaries. The definitions were completely tautological: the dictionary had defined disease in terms of symptoms and symptoms in terms of disease. It was like defining a term like "acrobat" as a person who performs "acrobatics" and then defining "acrobatics" as the activity performed by an "acrobat." If I didn't know one term, I couldn't know the other.

As far as I could tell, moreover, the term "disease" was a lot more complicated than the dictionary implied. In fact, my doctoral work in the history of medicine confirmed what these examples suggested: a disease is not a fixed entity defined for all time, but a useful classification dependent on society. While today we have an easy time classifying infectious diseases by referring to their dictionary definitions, other conditions prove more problematic. New experience may dictate that what we once thought of as a symptom should now be called a disease or vice versa; alternatively, what one culture considers a disease may be considered a quite normal event in another; and, finally, what at one time was a completely nonmedical state can by consensus become a disease.

So, what did it mean to call something a disease? I still didn't know, but I did know enough to slam the dictionary shut in exasperation.

I was not so naïve, of course, to assume that the answers to all questions come out of dictionaries, but they certainly weren't coming out of doctors or researchers either. Asking the meaning of medical terms was simply not something most medical professionals did. I couldn't imagine anyone standing up in the middle of a meeting, for example, to say, "Wait a second here. We've got to go back to square one and see if we all have the same understanding of what it means to call something a 'disease.'"

Few raise this question—either in medical schools or in medical meetings—because almost everyone outside of academic circles assumes that "we know what a disease is." Nor do most clinicians question their assumptions when they label two different patients as having the same specific disease. Like me, they generally assume that it's easy enough to look up specific diseases in a medical textbook or to look up the definition of "disease" in a medical dictionary. And, anyway, everyone knows the difference between a disease and a symptom—just consider measles and fever, for example. As I had discovered, however, we don't know.

In geometry, at some point in every analysis, people stop defining and rely on axioms—givens—which everyone is assumed to accept. Likewise, in most of the medical research I see, diseases are treated as axioms: rarely is there any effort to define either what a disease is in general, what the characteristics of a specific disease might be, or what makes a patient's condition a full-fledged "disease" rather than merely one or more "symptoms."

Few medical scientists or doctors think about disease conceptually. Thinking about fundamental medical concepts simply isn't a standard part of medical training or practice: doctors have to care for patients, analyze test results, and study for board examinations; scientists have to apply for grants, recalibrate thermometers, and supervise graduate students. Few have time to go back to first base and cross-examine medicine's traditional vocabulary.

The result is a pervasive problem for both medical science and medical practice. Much research loses significance because it can't be related to other research, and many patients receive improper care because their conditions are mislabeled. Again, none of this stems from evil doctors or incompetent scientists: it's just that everyone's talking about something different.

Debating the differences among "disease," "defect," "disorder," "symptom," "syndrome," and "illness" may seem like a needlessly theoretical and nitpickety attempt to define terms everybody knows— imperfectly, perhaps, but sufficiently for practical purposes.[6] The seemingly trivial and obvious, though, can sometimes have hidden and vital consequences. Making a formal (and vague) distinction between "disease" and "symptom" does not matter as much as recognizing the limitations inherent in the very notion of *distinct* diseases ("*definite* morbid processes"). The characteristics of a disease are ephemeral and elusive, so that the phenomena grouped together as a distinct disease by one perceptive physician or culture might well be separated by another. Alternatively, two different societies might give the same disease name to two different sets of phenomena—which of course doesn't make the two sets any more alike.

The idea of "distinct" diseases makes it all too easy to think that Real Diseases are hanging fully formed in the air, ready to fall on their unlucky victims. Like any abstract model of reality, this belief often helps us predict or explain events. But the transitoriness of our definitions—so bound to a particular time or place—should make us wary of taking for granted any definition or label of a disease, let alone assuming its concrete existence.

In this book I argue that unless we start asking ourselves what it really means to have a disease, the causes of disease will often remain elusive, prognoses uncertain, and therapies inappropriate. Unless investigators ask themselves this question, they will conduct shoddy research, one study irrelevant to the next. Unless physicians ask this question, they will mislead patients, misclassifying symptoms or belittling suffering. And unless patients ask this question, they will be confused and frustrated when they can't tag a name on their complaints.

Specifically, this book examines what happens when we don't define what we mean by a disease and when we prematurely define certain conditions as diseases. While exploring what it means for a group of conditions to be called a "disease," I discuss historical classifications that differ from today's as well as many conditions that still baffle medicine. These latter conditions provide a concrete opportunity to observe an ongoing historical transition—a movement from regarding phenomena as random symptoms to their naming as a formal disease. At such times what some people call a disease, others call a symptom or an imaginary event, and the contradictions among researchers and doctors multiply accordingly; thus, times of transition can damage both medical research and patient care. My hope is that by recognizing themselves as part of this ongoing historical process, all people whose illnesses fall between the cracks of currently recognized diseases will find some relief from their anxiety, frustration, and fear.

CHAPTER 1

Having an "In" Disease

▲ WHAT DO I HAVE, DOC?

Almost everyone who has ever felt ill—whether many nightly aches or several itchy spots or one sharp pain—has wondered, "What do I have? What is it?" We are frustrated at having an unexplained ailment and curse "the medical profession" when countless pokings and probings only lead the doctor to say, "You have a stomachache"—something we knew all along.

Our reasons for wanting a name attached to our ailments are largely unconscious and, in some ways, irrational. There is a part of us that doesn't want to know, after all, and we often prefer to think of a pain as a meaningless and transitory inconvenience. The man who feels dizzy, for example, would rather tell himself that he is tired than go in for a CAT scan and hear he has a brain tumor. With a little more sleep, he thinks, he will feel better.

Closer examination, however, shows that this man's first impulse on discovering a symptom (dizziness), the first thing he did to comfort himself, was to come up with an explanation and a course of action: he is dizzy *because* he is tired, and for relief he will sleep. Perhaps we wouldn't call "being tired" a disease; but it is certainly a distinct, generalized condition with associated symptoms, cause, and cure. For many, as we shall see, this is, or serves the same function as, a disease.

Our impulse, then, is to fit our complaints into larger patterns. We want to know why we feel bad so that we can eliminate the cause and feel better. This leads us to a basic principle of medical practice, although it is not always possible to apply the principle: one of the best ways to alleviate a problem is to alleviate its cause. For many established diseases, the patterns are known. Thus, if you look up the disease "tetanus" in the *Merck Manual* (a frequently used guide to medical diagnosis and treatment), you will find a technical description of that disease's "etiology," or set of causes: "Tetanus is caused by an exotoxin . . . elaborated by *Clostridium tetani,* a slender, motile, gram-positive, anaerobic, sporulating bacillus. The spores remain viable for years. . . . Tetanus may follow trivial as well as overtly contaminated wounds. . . . Drug addicts particularly are prone to develop tetanus. . . . Clinical disease does not confer immunity." Under the same heading, you will also find a description of the therapy for tetanus: "Therapy involves maintaining an adequate airway; early and adequate use of human immune serum globulin; neutralizing nonfixed toxin; preventing further toxin production; sedation; controlling muscle spasm, hypertonicity, fluid balance, and intercurrent infection; and continuous nursing care."[1]

By placing our aches and pains into the appropriate category, moreover, we also put an end to a frightening and infinite array of possibilities. The man with dizzy spells, for example, might comfort himself with the tiredness explanation for a while, but after getting more sleep and still feeling dizzy, he will begin to wonder. "Perhaps I'm not sleeping soundly," "Perhaps I'm sleeping too much," "Perhaps it's not sleep at all, but too much coffee." "Perhaps I'm allergic to my office furniture. I only seem to feel dizzy at work." "Come to think of it, maybe it's the stress at work." "Or maybe it's my heart. I've noticed irregular heartbeats now and then. Could circulation problems be cutting off the oxygen supply to my brain and making me dizzy?" "Is my posture wrong?" "Do I have a brain tumor?" "Am I crazy?" These questions go on and on, taking up more of the man's time and frightening him as the more innocuous possibilities prove unlikely. Perhaps he is in need of radiotherapy and is letting himself die by avoiding medical diagnosis. By learning the truth—even if it is the dreaded cancer—at least he knows what his chances are and can take some sort of action.[2]

Most people, then, find something comforting in knowing the name of their condition. My editor's eleven-year-old exclaimed happily when her knee pains were diagnosed as Osgood-Schlatter disease (a disorder, common in young adolescents, that involves pain, swelling, and tenderness at the end of the shinbone): "At least this time I've got

something with a name!" A friend of mine even says that he felt consid-
erable excitement when his doctor suggested that his bronchial problems might be due to Legionnaire's disease. Frightening as this disease
might be, at least having it would mean that his ills were legitimate and
that he could now take action. No one wants a disease, of course, but it
is far better to have a disease than merely to "feel bad."

▲ GRANTS, DRGs, AND PREMATURE NAMING

The pressure to name the thousands of human complaints does
not come only from patients in search of a label. Practicing physicians
as well as investigators are sometimes tempted to name illnesses as
diseases prematurely and to assign these names to individual patients
before there is an adequate way to distinguish the named condition
from other related conditions. Practitioners in particular know that the
right label can mean financial reward. As George Bernard Shaw pointed
out years ago, in his preface to *The Doctor's Dilemma,* "private medical
practice is governed not by science but by supply and demand. . . . [A]
serious illness or a death advertizes [sic] a doctor exactly as a hanging
advertizes the barrister who defended the person hanged." It is simply
more lucrative—not to mention more interesting—to treat a person
with a known disease than to proclaim ignorance and send her out the
door.[3] If you have diagnosed someone as having a rare and difficult
condition, you are a hero; if you simply say that you don't know what's
wrong and can't do anything about it, you lose not only one patient but
all those she may refer to you. In the medical economics of present-day
America, moreover, the federal government's diagnosis-related groups
(DRGs) mean that not labeling a patient optimally can undercut a hospital's reimbursement. Insurance companies differentially reimburse
different diseases, and in the event of uncertainty, a savvy doctor may
choose a more lucrative diagnosis.[4]

The fact is that not giving a name to a patient's complaint can
mean a disgruntled patient, a lack of financial compensation for your
time and effort, and perhaps even a malpractice suit. In fact, "failure
to diagnose" ranks at the top of malpractice claims against American
physicians.[5] Not surprisingly, then, many doctors feel pressured into
naming baffling conditions—or dismissing them altogether as "nothing"—rather than acknowledging the illness and simply admitting: "I
don't know what you have."

Scientists are equally eager to assign specific labels to a collection of isolated events and also often assign names to conditions prematurely. Scientists cannot do valid studies, after all, by looking only at individual cases. They must study a general phenomenon, or there will be too small a sample for statistically significant results. Thus, it is better to study "women with premenstrual syndrome" than to study "Elsie with anxiety five days before her period," "Janet with chocolate cravings one week a month," and "Rebecca with suicidal impulses at regular intervals."

In addition, the grants supporting most investigators these days are structured around specific diseases. It is easier to apply for funds if you are studying an entity such as "sickle-cell anemia" or "dyslexia" (especially if that entity is in vogue and well funded); simply puttering around in "inherited blood disorders" or "learning difficulties" will not get you a grant.

▲ KEEPING THE RIGHT COMPANY

Actually, it's not enough to have just any disease; it's crucial to have the *right* disease. In recent years, slick public relations firms and savvy lobbyists have produced a milieu in which diseases come in and out of fashion like hemlines. And if you're lucky enough to have an "in" disease, at least some of your suffering eases up: you know that you are not alone, that you have something real, and that you have a legitimate medical complaint that is not your fault.

"In" Diseases
Whatever the explanation, these "in" diseases are the ones nearly everyone—even people who know nothing about medicine—worry about, for their own sake or the world's. Being "in" has nothing to do with the seriousness or severity of the disease—even a condition as life-threatening as AIDS could be considered "in"—but rather with the degree of recognition and sympathy that sufferers from the disease can expect to receive. A disease can become "in" if a celebrity latches on to it, if a minority group protests loudly enough, or if a food industry decides its products will cure it. The idea of an "in" disease always makes me think back to the year I was twelve and crying my eyes out for braces on my teeth so that I could be "like everybody else." Somehow the pain didn't seem to matter very much, so long as I had company.

Of course, most "in" diseases are much more serious and unpleasant than braces. In the past few years, for example, osteoporosis (a degenerative disease of the bones) has become an "in" disease—television commercials tell you how to preserve your bone mass by exercising and by eating dairy foods, subway posters ask you to pity an elderly woman bent over with the condition, and cereal boxes promise super-high calcium levels that will prevent demineralization. Sickle-cell anemia has become an "in" disease, too, as have hypertension and muscular dystrophy (with its own telethon). Again, I am not saying that having an "in" disease is a desirable thing; it is still better to be healthy.

As gruesome as it is to have any disease, though, the truth remains: society is easier on you if it recognizes your disease. For one thing, there is a pretty good chance that if you have an "in" disease, someone else does, too—and suddenly there is peer support for what you once thought was your own miserable and lonely fate that no one, anywhere, could understand. Perhaps you will be able to join a group of people with similar problems; these support groups spring up readily whenever diseases happen to become "in." Since the late nineteenth century, doctors and laypeople have formed local and national societies to study, publicize, and treat some of these diseases; in recent years, moreover, groups hoping to publicize the "nameless diseases" have improved their tactics in an effort to assure victims as well as doctors that these unrecognized diseases are indeed real. The propaganda techniques of such organizations may be facilitating a process that in earlier times took decades, even centuries, to complete.

Through such organizations, people who have found a name for their suffering can read literature about others with the same disease or even attend meetings or classes with sympathizers. Patients with AIDS, for example, can choose from among community hospitals offering specially trained counselors, referral centers offering recommendations, and hotlines offering instant advice and support. Today there are support groups and associations for those with learning disabilities, dyslexia, endometriosis, puerperal mental illness, cerebral palsy, interstitial cystitis, premenstrual syndrome, Marfan syndrome, systemic lupus erythematosus, amyotrophic lateral sclerosis (Lou Gehrig's disease), epilepsy, multiple sclerosis, hearing problems, ileitis, colitis, coronary disease, diabetes, cancer, leukemia, scoliosis, muscular dystrophy, chronic fatigue syndrome, Tay-Sachs disease, sickle-cell anemia, Sjögren's syndrome, cystic fibrosis, Huntington's disease—the list could go on for pages.

On a lesser scale, the recent Orphan Drug Act makes some previously neglected diseases economically "in." Before the passage of this 1983 federal act, it was simply not cost-effective for drug companies to investigate therapies for such relatively rare diseases as Wilson's disease, an inherited condition in which the body cannot properly metabolize copper, and interstitial cystitis, a painful bladder disorder. The Orphan Drug Act has raised the status of these diseases by guaranteeing developers of "orphan drugs" (i.e., drugs aimed at potential patient populations of fewer than 200,000 people) seven years of market exclusivity and a 50 percent tax credit for certain clinical research expenses. People with orphan diseases may still have a hard time finding sympathy or even finding physicians to name their conditions; but once they do, they now have a chance to find treatment.[6]

Rett Syndrome

By reaching out to sufferers in a systematic fashion, support organizations are uniting people who in previous centuries might have spent entire lifetimes without finding support—or, in the case of what I call "nameless diseases," without even finding names for their ailment. For example, a reporter in Rhode Island told me about a woman named Carol Galuszka who spent twenty years baffled and guilty about the inexplicable behavior of her oldest daughter, Tammy.[7] Tammy acted like a normal child until she was about two years old, but suddenly everything seemed to fall apart. She started clenching one of her fists, staring off into space, and grimacing awkwardly. As Tammy grew older, she began wringing her hands almost constantly, withdrew emotionally, grew slowly, and never learned the basic skills of life.

At first, Carol was told that her daughter was autistic because she had been abused; later, other doctors decided that, no, Tammy wasn't autistic: she was mentally retarded. And yet, it didn't make sense. If this child was really "just retarded," then why had she been such a normal baby? Why was she so thin despite all the food she ate? And why did she wring her hands like that? In any case, since she had ceased to be officially "autistic" and had become "mentally retarded," she was forced to withdraw from her school, a school designed for autistic children.

Only when Tammy was a young woman did her mother discover the answer. Reading a newsletter published by a society on autism, she learned about another little girl who had been mistakenly diagnosed as autistic but who actually had a little-known condition called Rett syndrome. Often mistaken for autism or mental retardation, Rett syndrome was actually a disease all its own, with its own set of characteristics. Immediately, Carol knew that "Rett syndrome" was the name she had been searching for all these years.

For the one out of every ten thousand or so females who develops this syndrome, babyhood appears normal, but at about age two something happens: basic skills fall off, and a temporary period of autistic behavior usually follows. Girls with Rett syndrome are known for their compulsive handwringing, stiff-legged walk, facial grimaces, teeth-grinding, seizures, spasticity, poor leg circulation, severe to profound retardation, and, in later years, abnormally small heads and curved spines. Clearly then, labeling girls with these features as "autistic" or "mentally retarded" is inaccurate. Rett syndrome is a condition all its own, and behaviors that seem autistic or mentally retarded are just symptoms of it.

But Carol Galuszka couldn't have learned about this syndrome until a little organizational networking had set the stage. Although Dr. Andreas Rett himself, a rather obscure Viennese practitioner, had described this syndrome more than a decade earlier, no one had paid much attention. Only in 1983, with the help of a prominent Swedish neurologist did the word of this syndrome reach the international medical press, and that was enough to start the ball rolling.[8] Once the condition had an officially recognized name, doctors began organizing international conferences, which attracted eminent scientists, doctors, and researchers; suddenly observations from all over the world magnified the experience of one doctor. It was only natural that a support organization would follow, and in early 1985 the International Rett Syndrome Association was born.

With this formal organization in place, life would never be the same for the families of girls with Rett syndrome. The woman who had written the newsletter article on the syndrome had been lucky enough to have a doctor active in the International Rett Syndrome Association. It was also lucky that an autism organization existed to publish a newsletter. Her article alerted the many people who had lived for years in ignorance of their daughters' condition; it gave them the name they had been searching for. This name also offered a realistic hope for effective treatment: before anyone had recognized Rett syndrome as a distinct disease, of course, there could be no one studying it. More concretely, a strong association helped encourage the funding so vital to effective research. Testimony from the newly formed International Rett Syndrome Association, in fact, persuaded the U.S. Congress to appropriate $500,000 for Rett syndrome research to the National Institute of Child Health and Human Development. Further testimony not only led the National Institute of Neurological and Communicative Disorders and Stroke to send their chief of developmental neurology (the person who decides which research projects to fund) to the 1986 International Conference on Rett Syndrome, but in 1989 also resulted in funding for two multimillion-dollar research projects.

All this meant that once Carol Galuszka opened that autism newsletter, she was quickly able to accomplish more than she had over the past twenty years. As she read the article, she realized that her family was no longer alone. She immediately wrote to the president of the International Rett Syndrome Association, and he invited her to the next conference. There she met Dr. Rett and had Tammy's condition confirmed. She also took home a handbag full of brochures and other literature on Rett syndrome that the association had published, and she distributed this information to Tammy's doctors and teachers back home. Hastening medical progress even more, she sent information on the little-known syndrome to every local pediatrician, just to make sure that no other little girl went as long as Tammy Galuszka had without a name for her disease.

Einstein Had Dyslexia, You Know

Other organizations go further than just providing a name and sympathy. They actually boost the egos of disease victims by citing famous people who suffered from the same maladies—vaguely implying that anyone who has this disease may actually be a little "better" than people without it. The logic here is questionable, but the efficacy undeniable: people like to think that they share something, even if it is a disease, with someone great. Thus, using evidence sometimes tenuous at best, two authors writing about premenstrual syndrome (PMS) cite an impressive array of women who are known to have shown erratic, irrational, and volatile behaviors—including Mary Todd Lincoln, Sylvia Plath, Maria Callas, Queen Victoria, Pauline Bonaparte, Alice James, Judy Garland, Catherine of Aragon, Mary Tudor, and even Elizabeth I— and suggest that they may have had PMS.[9] Although recognizing the difficulty of proving such claims—it is extremely doubtful that any of these women kept rigorous records of their behavior in correlation with their menstrual cycles (especially before anyone knew anything about PMS) or that these records would have survived even if they ever existed—the authors insist countless times that these women may well have had PMS and would have been so diagnosed if only the medical profession had been aware of PMS in their day. Yes, indeed, they may, but why devote a significant portion of a book to developing a hypothesis with virtually no evidence? Clearly because it makes readers who think they have "PMS" feel better to know that they are among greats.

Occasionally, of course, there may be an actual link between a disease and greatness or talent. People with dyslexia, for example, show no obvious physical or mental handicaps but, despite an adequate social and educational environment, have a special difficulty with language. Although it is not yet known whether the combination of problems called dyslexia is caused by some identifiable brain defect, it is conceivable that whatever produces dyslexia may at the same time enhance other skills—perhaps mathematical or artistic ones—just as the same gene responsible for sickle-cell anemia protects an individual against malaria. Thus, in a great deal of the literature on this condition, victims are told that fellow sufferers may well have included Leonardo da Vinci, Michelangelo, Auguste Rodin, William Butler Yeats, Hans Christian Andersen, Agatha Christie, Thomas Edison, George Patton, Winston Churchill, Woodrow Wilson, Nelson Rockefeller, and even Albert Einstein.

To a child feeling stupid because of his troubles learning to read, inclusion in such a group of luminaries certainly couldn't hurt. Of course, just because Albert Einstein may have had dyslexia but was also a genius does not mean that every little Billy who can't learn to read is also a genius. But it certainly makes him proud to know that he has the same "disease" as Einstein.

Puerperal Mental Illness

Having a disease with some "physical or biochemical cause," however serious, is also often preferable to having what many people may regard as a vague psychological "problem." Consider a thirty-two-year-old woman who has just given birth to her first child. Three days after the delivery, she becomes restless and irritable and then suddenly depressed and exhausted. She also feels weak, sweats heavily, and has trouble sleeping, but she decides she must still be getting over the trauma of the delivery. A few days later, though, she becomes suspicious of everyone around her, mumbles incoherently about dreams and deformities, worries that she might hurt her baby, and generally acts irrationally. Another week goes by and her husband finds her about to break the baby's arm with her bare hands.

Now, when this woman first can't bring herself to get out of bed to pick up her screaming newborn, she may suspect that her problems are caused by some physical illness. This suspicion will naturally worry her, and the next morning she may ask her doctor for an explanation. But, as James Alexander Hamilton, a psychiatrist specializing in similar problems following childbirth, has pointed out, if a well-meaning doctor "reassures" this woman that there is no physical cause for her feelings, her anxiety may mount.[10] Told that "nothing" is causing her problems, the new mother may fear that incompetence, failure as a woman, or insanity underlies her symptoms. Ironically, these fears may well provoke or aggravate some real psychiatric illness, resulting in delirium and violence.

What the woman's doctor could have told her, however, was that such problems can often appear several days following a delivery, even if the new mother has never had any mental health problems before. He could have told her that a growing number of doctors might suspect "puerperal mental illness" (puerperal means following birth)—which, according to some psychiatrists, is a very different kind of mental illness than standard "schizophrenia" or "manic-depressive disorder."

According to these same psychiatrists, this sort of misnaming occurs more often than not among modern doctors. Ironically, until the late nineteenth century, doctors acknowledged that the mental illness following childbirth was a special kind of disease and treated patients accordingly; then, more "sophisticated" psychiatrists decided that the term "puerperal mental illness" was meaningless and dropped it from the psychiatric literature. Only in the past decade or so have some doctors tried to revive the term and reeducate the rest of their profession.

Although doctors still don't know exactly what causes this condition, most of those who believe it exists as a specific disease suspect that it has something to do with the drastic changes in hormone levels following a birth; when these adjust back to normal, the woman behaves much as she did before the pregnancy. Thus, if this condition is caused by some temporary hormonal imbalance, it can be treated medically. Quite clearly, then, when a doctor tells a new mother that she has "puerperal mental illness"—something with a biochemical explanation—she is going to feel a lot less upset than she would if he told her she was a crazy or inept woman who had "rejected her maternal feelings."[11] By receiving a medical name for her condition, a name that implies a biochemical imbalance, the new mother is able to believe that, through no fault of her own, she has a disease and that medical care will keep her under control.

A name that implies a physical problem is best not only for your own peace of mind, but for your social status as well. Society at large is much more kindly disposed toward a person with a physical problem than toward one who is either evil, stupid, or crazy; in fact, our society generally blames people who can't attribute their suffering to a germ or a fall or a chemical imbalance.[12]

▲ THE WRONG COMPANY

Of course, even "in" diseases can have devastating social consequences. In fact, many support groups have arisen in order to combat the preexisting stigmas that various diseases carry. Recent publicity about the AIDS label—children banned from school, workers fired from jobs, friends shunned by friends—is only an extreme version of the stigma attached to many disease names. Thus, people generally don't like to be told that they have had an "epileptic seizure," for they sense an unspoken societal fear of people with epilepsy, especially the fear that it is related in some way to mental illness.[13] Similarly, in the 1960s, the name "autism" applied to a child was associated with neglectful, abusive parents. And the chronic condition gout, nothing more than a form of arthritis often caused by crystallized uric acid that has built up in the joints, long had the reputation of being specifically caused by (sinful) overindulgence in rich food and alcohol.[14]

Often these stigmas carry over into a sufferer's livelihood. In fact, a recent *Wall Street Journal* article observes that "illness-related" job discrimination is common and likely to rise as more seriously ill people survive and as "AIDS continues its onslaught."[15] This article tells the story of a twenty-six-year-old undercover vice cop in New York City who had suffered from a form of cancer called lymphoma. After eight months of intermittent hospitalization, radiation, and chemotherapy, however, she was pronounced in remission and returned to her job. Just a few months later, her superior called her into his office to announce that "Headquarters" had phoned and that she was being terminated immediately—despite the fact that she had been making more arrests than most of her colleagues, sick or well, male or female. The reason? She had "cancer."

"Having cancer makes you feel abnormal to begin with," the policewoman was quoted as saying. "There's a stigma. People make you feel different. I was just getting back to feeling normal. Then, they tried to put that stigma back on me. I had to fight."

This reaction is not unlike that of parents who learn that their children have a "learning disability." Although their first reaction may be relief that their suspicions have been confirmed, quite soon afterward their response is "amazement, shock, disbelief, and especially anger—at the teacher, the school, and particularly the child," reports Betty Osman in her book on learning disabilities. They start seeing their child as "less mature, less competent, and surely less successful," even observing that the child "'looked different,' resembling for the first time that black sheep brother or other unsuccessful relative whom no one mentions anymore."[16]

These views can actually influence the patients themselves, as sort of self-fulfilling prophesies. One psychiatrist at a meeting of the Orton Dyslexia Society said that he liked to use the term "dyslexia" instead of "learning disabled," because he had found that kids labeled as "learning disabled" tended to be depressed and suicidal. He believed that, just by changing the name, he could change the nature of the disease.

On the other hand, the name "dyslexia" has its own set of bad associations. David Jobson wrote in the *British Medical Journal* that dyslexia still "has a slightly dirty name." He recalls that in 1976, when he was training in pediatrics, his consultant taught him "that the word was a useful dumping ground for middle class families who need an excuse for the poor performance in school of their not very intelligent children." Thus, when his own nine-year-old daughter developed reading and disciplinary problems characteristic of dyslexia, he preferred to think of her as "undisciplined" rather than use the term "dyslexia."[17]

Reasons for the stigmas attached to certain conditions, including—but not restricted to—cancer, heart trouble, epilepsy, premenstrual syndrome, diabetes, autism, dyslexia, and AIDS are many and complex. Some are partially justifiable in that they are related to increased insurance costs and to fears that the employee will take too many sick days. Others, however, are the result of an unfounded fear of contagion. Still others are more subtle and relate to an unconscious dislike of the weak or a generalized fear of mortality.

In some workplaces, notably those which receive money from the U.S. government, "labeled" workers who can really do their job may be able to get their fair economic share through the Rehabilitation Act of 1973. But even the most promising of laws cannot end the humiliation and social stigmas that many disease names engender. The *Wall Street Journal* describes a gardener who had worked for San Francisco's Parks and Recreation Department for more than a year and who had received excellent performance reviews. By accident, his supervisor learned that he wore an eyepatch because he once had eye cancer. He fired the worker. True, the gardener was rehired after filing a complaint with the city, but the stigma lived on. People who have recovered from heart attacks and have gone through rehabilitation programs, even when they are in better health than ever before, face similar problems.

Having a name also means that you take on a preset pattern that may not be applicable to you as an individual. Several years ago, for example, a Manhattan artist in her early thirties developed swollen glands in her throat and neck. Months of painful examination and testing procedures revealed that she had "lymphoma," and further tests were then performed to determine the exact type of lymphoma. "I knew in the back of my mind that lymphoma was 'cancer,'" she said, "but I couldn't use that word. I felt better telling my friends that I have this obscure condition that they had never heard of—lymphoma—and describing what it involved, than saying, or admitting to myself, that I had cancer. Having cancer is being dead."

Thus, by avoiding a particular name, "cancer," she could go on living and did not have to associate herself with all the painful and gruesome cancer deaths she had read about—and perhaps rightfully so, for her course of treatment and outcome were successful. At present, she appears to be cured and has returned to her work.

Many other diseases are associated with similar mythologies that automatically attach to any of the sufferers. For example, endometriosis has a reputation for being "the career woman's disease," afflicting working women in their late twenties and early thirties who have not "stopped to have children"—a label that frustrates women with endometriosis who do have babies, not to mention teenagers with the condition. Black women with endometriosis are likewise frustrated by the common notion that endometriosis is rare among blacks. At the same time, even childless, white working women who do fit the stereotype resent the implication that they are somehow to blame for their pain. All of these women resent being thought of as "nervous" and "overanxious," terms also commonly associated with endometriosis.[18]

▲ GETTING THE RIGHT CARE

Does it really matter if we say a sick patient has a specific disease or not? As we have just seen, psychologically it may matter a great deal to the patient. Patients come to doctors expecting a name for what is "wrong" with them and feel dissatisfied if they leave without one.[19] Once we can attach a name to our illness, after all, we can fit ourselves into a very specific niche; this alleviates fears of even worse conditions, tells us what we can expect, and gives us faith that the doctor can choose an appropriate course of action. At the same time, some names carry stigmas with them, making it even more important for patients to make sure that the name they have been assigned really "belongs" to them.

A specific disease label can also make a tremendous difference in the way a doctor deals with a patient. When a doctor diagnoses a specific disease, he is saying that the patient's symptoms or lab results or genetic structure or personal habits or whatever fit into a predetermined pattern. This pattern may be a simple, common etiology or a complex laundry list of vague feelings. Appropriate treatment will hinge on which pattern the doctor pinpoints.

Consider a common wart and a form of skin cancer called squamous-cell carcinoma, for example. To an untrained eye, these two conditions may look very similar: both can involve a firm lump on the skin that looks something like a small cauliflower, but doctors distinguish the two because each condition represents a different pattern; each is associated with a different "cause" as well as a different "prognosis." Specifically, while the wart is linked to a virus and may well disappear naturally without any untoward effects, the carcinoma is probably the result of cell damage (perhaps by sunlight) and may spread to other parts of the body, occasionally even causing death. Consequently, the common wart and the squamous-cell carcinoma require different care, and if a patient receives the wrong name for his disease, he will receive inappropriate therapy.

Some diseases are recognized as distinct patterns because they have different biochemical or mechanical roots. In these cases, treatment depends on removing or remedying the root, making an appropriate name all the more crucial. Both the neurological conditions myasthenia gravis and Bell's palsy involve weakened facial muscles, for example, but they are treated quite differently. In myasthenia gravis, the characteristic muscle fatigue seems to be related to low levels of the neurotransmitter acetylcholine and a consequent impairment of the facial muscles' ability to contract. Thus, treatment of myasthenia gravis primarily involves drugs that boost the body's supply of acetylcholine. In contrast, facial paralysis in Bell's palsy stems from a swollen, pinched nerve, and so treatment generally involves protecting the exposed eye (usually using eyedrops or a temporary patch) and then administering drugs to decompress the facial nerve.

Even related diseases require correct naming if patients are to expect appropriate treatment. Consider the condition "epilepsy." Although many laypeople regard it as a single disease—and, indeed, any kind of epilepsy involves some kind of "seizure" in which the neurons of the brain fire inappropriately—epileptic seizures can vary greatly in character. In petit mal epilepsy, which is almost always limited to children, seizures begin and end abruptly. From ten to fifty times a day, the child will stop whatever he is doing and stare, growing pale; he may flutter his eyelids and drop his head slightly forward. But he does not fall on the floor in the uncontrollable twitches associated with stereotypical epilepsy; in fact, he usually remains seated, and no one may even notice anything amiss. These seizures occur all over the brain, not in one particular area.

Another form of epilepsy, known as the partial seizure, can look very similar. Here the patient has hardly noticeable lapses of consciousness or suddenly begins to suck, chew, or swallow. Proper diagnosis is crucial, because although partial seizures can look very much like petit mal seizures, these two forms of epilepsy involve different brain patterns and require very different treatment. Thus, the drug primidone is a fairly effective drug for partial seizures but is useless in treating petit mal seizures.[20] A patient's health, then, depends on the doctor naming the patient's epilepsy correctly.

In other cases, patients may be able to *afford* care only if they get the right name. Especially since the advent of DRGs in the United States, government agencies and insurance companies allocate funds to individuals or hospitals according to the specific diseases; patients with some diseases get more help than others, regardless of whether one person is sicker than another. In April 1986, for example, a little girl named Melanie Broderick was born in New Hampshire with an unidentifiable condition: two weeks after birth she arched her back and began screaming; she also stopped swallowing and developed other neurological problems. And although for the next five months Melanie's parents dragged her around to dozens of specialists on the East Coast—all of whom concluded that the child was screaming only because she had "colic"—at seventeen months (long after colic usually subsides) Melanie's problems had not diminished, and nobody could identify "what was wrong." Without a name to wave around, the child's parents couldn't get any help from a private charity or support group targeted to some specific disease. Furthermore, because an undiagnosed condition can't be called permanent, they were barred from Social Security benefits earmarked for the "permanently disabled."[21]

Yet, even a diagnosis can prevent benefits by excluding the sick person from a fundable category. Until recently, for example, people who had the condition then known as AIDS-related complex (ARC) were not eligible for the automatic disability benefits given to people with the similar disease AIDS. ARC had no clear-cut definition but generally referred to people who had antibodies to the AIDS virus in their blood and had some of the milder symptoms of AIDS without any lethal opportunistic infections (such as Kaposi's sarcoma or pneumocystis pneumonia). ARC victims were known to die from their condition, though, and most suffered from severe weight loss, swollen glands, high fever, chronic diarrhea, dementia, fatigue, and night sweats. In fact, some researchers were beginning to suspect that ARC might be some form of "pre-AIDS."

Because ARC was then considered a separate disease, however, it had a different funding status than AIDS. In fact, although there were many more ARC patients than AIDS patients, and although some people with ARC were sicker than those with AIDS, only "AIDS" was listed among those diseases which automatically qualified a patient for disability benefits. People with ARC were also much less likely to be at the top of a doctor's list for an experimental drug treatment that was designated for "AIDS victims."[22]

In short, the definition of "ARC" did not have enough in common with the definition of "AIDS" to fit into the latter category. And so, if you had ARC, you suffered the same stigma as someone with AIDS—where did you get that virus, people wondered—and your symptoms were often as severe, but you didn't get any of the benefits. You couldn't get health care from clinics that helped only "AIDS" victims, and you couldn't join support groups for AIDS victims either. Nonetheless, eventually you may well have developed full-blown AIDS anyway. That's why some epidemiologists started to wonder whether people with ARC might not belong in the AIDS category after all—just as we are apt to say that someone with a cold virus and the sniffles has a cold. They had the virus, after all, and they may have gone on to develop symptoms of the full-blown disease. Some doctors therefore strove to change the definition of AIDS to include ARC so that ARC victims could get health care from those agencies which then offered help only for official "AIDS" patients.[23]

This concern for getting the right name assigned to an illness may seem simpleminded, especially since there are a fair number of diseases that we have no problem defining; in particular, diseases associated with a microorganism are usually not confused. We basically know that measles is different from diphtheria is different from syphilis is different from mumps, and we very rarely confuse one with another. But for many other medical conditions, as we shall see, it is not always so easy to get the name right.

CHAPTER 2

▲

Having a "Nameless" Disease

Ellie, Tommy, and Gail have very little in common.[1] Ellie is a fifty-six-year-old executive secretary who enjoys musical comedy and Thai food; Tommy is an earnest eight-year-old schoolboy who builds model airplanes in his free time; and Gail is a thirty-five-year-old piano teacher and the mother of two school-age children. But although their lives and concerns overlap very little, all three do have one thing in common: they all have nameless diseases.

Ellie's troubles began two years ago when she was fifty-four. She began to feel a disturbing pressure on her bladder as if she had to urinate. She felt this pressure almost all the time—only urinating seemed to relieve it—and she found herself making constant trips to the ladies' room. She tried drinking less, but the problem only worsened. Going to the theater and out to dinner were embarrassing enough, but when she had to leave her desk every forty-five minutes during the day, she knew that she had a serious medical condition.

Ellie made an appointment with her family doctor the next week. This doctor listened patiently as she described her symptoms and then, suspecting that she probably had cystitis—an infection of the bladder—he tested her urine for bacteria. But when the test came back negative, the doctor told Ellie that there didn't seem to be a physical problem; if she just reduced the stress in her life, the pressure would go away. When Ellie protested, the doctor recommended a psychiatrist.

Tommy's troubles, on the other hand, started last year when he began having trouble in school. Although he had received top-notch instruction and always made A's in math, he could barely read. In fact, he could barely write the alphabet: his *b*'s looked like *d*'s sometimes, and his *u*'s looked like *n*'s. Tommy would also throw paper airplanes at his classmates while he was supposed to be studying and stare out the window when his teacher asked him a question.

Tommy's teacher suggested that he be kept back a grade until his reading picked up. She also noted in his record that he was a "discipline problem." Yet, a year later, neither Tommy's reading nor his behavior had improved, and there was talk of sending him to military school.

Finally, Gail, the piano teacher, had problems of her own. Most of the time she was a mild-mannered woman, happy listening to the neighborhood children practicing scales. But for about a week every month, right before her menstrual period, she would get a pounding headache and sense vague anger at the world. To make matters worse, she always gained five pounds at this time and her face broke out in a mess of acne, just as it had when she was fifteen. Feeling fat and ugly only made her angrier. Sometimes the anger would become so strong that she found herself screaming at little girls who missed a sharp or rapping the knuckles of little boys who forgot to bend their fingers.

When mothers started complaining, Gail decided to ask her gynecologist for help. But this doctor told her that there was nothing wrong that a little willpower couldn't take care of: Gail could take aspirin for the headaches, but she would just have to learn to control herself.

The frustrations of Ellie, Tommy, and Gail result from having conditions that have no well-defined, universally accepted labels. Because many doctors don't know what to call these nameless diseases, patients can spend painful years not knowing what they have—or thinking they have something they don't. Specifically, what Ellie's doctor called "stress" may well have been interstitial cystitis; what Tommy's teacher called a "discipline problem" may well have been dyslexia; and what Gail's doctor called a "lack of willpower" may well have been premenstrual syndrome.

▲ DISEASES WITHOUT NAMES

Unfortunately, doctors are still debating whether interstitial cystitis, dyslexia, and premenstrual syndrome—as well as many other nameless diseases—are true medical conditions at all. Until these debates are settled, patients like Ellie, Tommy, and Gail are going to suffer. In Chapter 1 we learned of similar suffering in people who couldn't find names—or the right names—for their diseases. The present chapter will help explain why finding names is so difficult for people with nameless diseases and how our society can allow all this needless guilt, pain, and frustration.

There is quite a large number of nameless diseases. These are often (but not always) chronic conditions that lack any universally accepted definition;[2] although they look like real diseases to some people, not everyone in the medical community will recognize them or even suspect that they exist. Consequently, while one doctor may name a nameless disease, another will say that the condition is simply imaginary or only a symptom of some other disease. Without the universal support of the medical community, getting friends and colleagues to believe that a nameless disease is a "real" medical condition can be even more frustrating.

I call such conditions "nameless" not because they don't ever have names, but because people who have these conditions may spend an inordinate amount of time not knowing what they have—or thinking they have something they don't.[3] What one doctor calls "seasonal affective disorder," for example, can be what other doctors regard as no disease at all but something attributable to moodiness or hypochondria; similarly, what one doctor calls "dysmenorrhea" can be what others regard not as a unique disease but as a run-of-the-mill neurosis that happens to peak during a woman's menstrual period.

The line between an "in" disease and a "nameless" disease can be extremely thin at times. In fact, once a nameless disease achieves full recognition, it can quickly become an "in" disease, especially if the same support groups that legitimized the disease continue to spread the word. Consider Lyme disease, a form of arthritis that sometimes results from the bite of a deer tick and that can affect many bodily systems, including the joints, the heart, and the brain. In the mid-1970s, Lyme disease was a nameless disease, and people suffering from it went from doctor to doctor without a diagnosis, often told that they were "hypochondriacs."[4] By the late 1980s, however, you could read about Lyme disease and how to prevent it in almost any major metropolitan newspaper. Premenstrual syndrome, too, hovers right now between the two worlds. For those people who "believe" that it is a distinct medical condition, PMS is definitely "in," and, as we shall see later in this book, even women who don't have the condition want to claim the name. On the other hand, for those people who still dismiss PMS as a flimsy excuse for moodiness, PMS remains as nameless as ever.

Conditions that are or once were nameless diseases include puerperal mental illness, AIDS-related complex, gestational diabetes, learning disability, Rett syndrome, seasonal affective disorder (SAD), chronic fatigue immune dysfunction syndrome (CFIDS), myalgic encephalomyelitis (ME), fibromyalgia, temporomandibular joint (TMJ) syndrome, Reye's (Reye) syndrome, Tourette syndrome, dysmenorrhea, Sjögren's syndrome, colic, sudden infant death syndrome ("crib death"), multiple sclerosis, chronic pain syndrome, labyrinthitis, Wilson's disease, microvascular angina ("syndrome X"), repetitive stress injury (RSI), migraine, and endometriosis. Even more pervasive, however, are all the nameless diseases that comprise the vague aches, pains, and spasms that everyone feels but no one can identify as part of a specific disease. Nameless diseases can involve all those feelings like sadness or apathy which many of us attribute to our own weakness or to "real" diseases like depression or heart disease but which may stem in some unclear way from our social and environmental setting—from loneliness, malnutrition, rejection, or lack of light, for example. Such nameless diseases exist not because doctors are ignorant, but simply because the vast majority of human complaints remain almost completely misunderstood: they cannot be linked with other conditions or traced to a specific cause; therefore, they cannot be categorized into our rather limited list of official diseases. From this perspective, there's probably no one on the planet who at one time or another hasn't experienced the symptoms of a nameless disease.

Skeptics may interject here that many people who have these nameless diseases are simply "malingerers" or "hypochondriacs" or that their symptoms are "psychosomatic." All of these terms are simply different ways of saying what people with nameless diseases hear all the time: "it's all in your head." In the popular parlance, all three of these accusations imply that if people with nameless diseases do suffer from anything "objective," that something is psychological rather than physical. Here I would agree that a small percentage of people who seem to have nameless diseases (as well as a small percentage of people who seem to have well-recognized diseases) may indeed be malingerers. That is to say, these people are purposely pretending to suffer in order to receive certain benefits that society confers upon the ill. Although these people deserve our sympathy and probably require some form of therapy, they cannot be considered to be true sufferers of nameless diseases.

On the other hand, there is no reason why suffering from hypochondria or psychosomatic illness precludes a person from having a nameless disease. Indeed, given the circumstances involving the search for a name, it would be surprising if these terms never applied. According to the psychologist Susan Baur, the term "hypochondria" simply refers to people who "unwittingly center their lives on health or disease and yet who function well enough to live in normal society." Such a focus may lead people with hypochondria to exaggerate the severity of symptoms, but being a hypochondriac does not per se exclude the possibility of having genuine physical problems. Likewise, people with psychosomatic illness by definition have genuine physical problems, but these problems are triggered, exacerbated, or maintained by some kind of "psychological stress."[5] It is possible to suffer from both hypochondria and psychosomatic illness simultaneously, moreover, and equally possible to suffer from either or both of these conditions and still have a nameless disease. After all, if you spend years searching for a name and are told repeatedly that nothing is wrong with you and that your pain is imaginary, it's not unlikely that you'll become "centered" on your physical state. Nor is it unlikely that the psychological stress resulting from such an experience will aggravate or sustain some of your original physical symptoms.

Thus, labeling people as "hypochondriacs" or their symptoms as "psychosomatic" is irrelevant to determining whether or not their condition can be attributed to a nameless disease. Furthermore, while it is likely that some people who attribute their symptoms to a nameless disease may indeed suffer from hypochondria, "hysteria" (conversion disorder), or somatization disorder (Briquet's syndrome), it is equally possible that other people diagnosed as suffering from these neurotic conditions (with their ever-shifting definitions) may actually have one of the nameless diseases.

However you (or others) label your psychological state, if you do have the symptoms of a nameless disease that at least potentially has a known name, you're probably anxious to have it assigned to you. The name a doctor assigns is not only going to make your symptoms seem "legitimate," but is going to affect the kind of treatment you get: a diagnosis of "dysmenorrhea" may get you a prescription for anti-inflammatory tablets, while the diagnosis of "hypochondria" may just get you scorn. An obstetrician ignorant of puerperal mental illness, for example, hardly atypical in this day and age, may well misdiagnose a woman with that nameless disease. Many doctors who would never dismiss the woman as a "bad mother" still do not recognize puerperal mental illness as a distinct medical entity—and some doctors have not even heard of it! They know about mental illness in general, but the fact that the mental illness occurred right after a pregnancy seems to them irrelevant in making a specific diagnosis.

A new mother classified as simply "depressed" and put in a ward with other mental patients may not realize that her kind of depression—postpartum—is of a very different sort from the depression of the woman in the next bed who has tried to kill herself five times. She may think her disease is long-term and that only years of pills and psychiatrists can restore her.[6]

Finding a name for your suffering can remove this sort of censure. Take Mrs. B., for example, a twenty-nine-year-old housewife from Westchester County, New York. Even as a young teenager, Mrs. B. felt irritable and agitated right before her period. At that time of the month, she'd develop an intermittent headache, painfully tender breasts, severe cramps, and pelvic discomfort—all topped off by a dark depression. But nobody could explain why this was happening to her. "I told my mother and my family physician when I was fifteen years old," she says, "and I told several doctors through the years. But no tests were done, and I just attributed symptoms to my 'time of the month.' I told myself that 'this was just me . . .' and that I should live with it." Apparently the doctors agreed with her: "All they said was to take Tylenol and bear with it. These doctors made me feel that I was a hypochondriac."

It was only eight years later, when Mrs. B. was twenty-three years old, that she read about PMS in a popular magazine and began to suspect that something physical might be wrong with her. It took several more painful appointments, but eventually she found a doctor who agreed. He diagnosed her as having PMS and suggested she try vitamin therapy. "Suddenly I felt like I had a real thing, and I wasn't just a hypochondriac," says Mrs. B, observing the difference she felt once her complaints had a name: "Everything suddenly changed. I think the doctors treated me differently once they realized that PMS is a condition in many women—not just me. Also, my family members now understand that I get irritable and sick temporarily and that it's not my fault." Having spoken with other women who also have PMS, Mrs. B. no longer has to feel that "it's just me."

A twenty-two-year-old nurse from a town in northern England ("C") had a similar experience. She began "feeling draggy" following any kind of exercise or mental exertion. When this fatigue went on for months, she went to see her general practitioner, who attributed her symptoms to "depression." Concerned about a depression so severe that it could fully exhaust her, C. checked herself into a mental hospital, where the doctors on staff prescribed antidepressants. Yet, C. didn't feel any more energetic; in fact, she found herself talking incredibly slowly. But since no one at the hospital could find a psychological or psychiatric explanation for her condition, they released her.

She kept getting worse. There were many days when she felt that she couldn't move at all. She felt so tired that she couldn't walk, talk, or eat, and sometimes she found herself shivering or sweating excessively. She was home alone, scared, and (not surprisingly) depressed. Fortuitously, during one of her particularly bad days, she forced herself to go see a couple from her church, and when she described her problems to them, they were struck by the familiarity of her story. The fatigue after exertion, the malaise, the sensitivity to extremes of temperature, the emotional lability—all of these symptoms sounded a lot like those of the husband, who had been diagnosed as having "myalgic encephalomyelitis," or ME.[7]

Recognized by only a small segment of physicians, ME is another nameless disease. Despite seventy or so suspected outbreaks, ME is often misdiagnosed as hysteria, depression, or hypochondria by doctors who would rather offer a name than admit ignorance. The young nurse, C., was lucky that her friends had a doctor who had actually heard of ME and believed that it was a "real" condition, possibly related to a viral infection and definitely not "all in the head." For the first time, C. says, someone reassured her that she was not just a weak woman.

"Having a name made a world of difference," C. continues. Now she can belong to the ME Association, an organization full of other people who understand why she feels the way she does. Now she can tell her coworkers why she's "draggy," and instead of belittling her they understand that she's the victim of this disease. "In fact," C. adds, "I doubt I could have kept my job if I hadn't had this name for my symptoms."

Even well-established diseases can sometimes change their form enough so that they temporarily become nameless. Poliomyelitis provides a particularly vivid example. This disease, known in the late nineteenth century by various names, including infantile paralysis, has probably existed since earliest civilization. Throughout most of its history, it afflicted mainly infants, occurring sporadically rather than in large epidemics. A baby would have a fever, and several days or weeks later parents would notice that the baby was lame. Sometimes they even attributed this lameness to teething and, hard as it is for many of us today to believe, accepted their child's fate as an unfortunate but inevitable accompaniment of some childhood fevers. Only in 1789 was this disease of infants even described with its own name in a medical text.

Then, in the late nineteenth century, doctors started to think they were seeing an entirely new disease, fundamentally distinct from this occasional paralysis of infants following fever. This "new" disease occurred in epidemics. It afflicted older children as well as infants. Doctors in the 1930s still thought that this disease came into being at the turn of the twentieth century, perhaps brought on by a new and more virulent strain of the virus associated with infantile paralysis. For doctors trained to think in terms of "infantile paralysis," however, patients with symptoms of this "new" disease often lived without diagnoses, like all patients with nameless diseases. In his history of poliomyelitis, the medical historian John R. Paul relates the story of a seventeen-year-old girl who was admitted to the adult medical service of the New Haven Hospital in June 1931, complaining of fever, drowsiness, back pain, and general weakness. No one knew what was wrong with her, though. She didn't seem to fit into any known categories, and yet she was clearly very ill. The answer came only later when the girl herself volunteered the information that she couldn't seem to move her legs. Although it wasn't polio season, and although polio in adolescents was rare, the girl did indeed have polio, as did many other adolescents in the 1931 epidemic that followed.[8] During World War II, U.S. Army physicians had similar troubles attaching disease names to the many sick soldiers stationed abroad who had symptoms of polio. They had been stationed in countries where polio was sporadic if it was noticed at all, and young adults weren't supposed to get polio anyway—certainly not in large outbreaks. And yet, it soon became clear that these young men, too, were suffering from polio.

The explanation, developed years later, depends on an understanding that polio results after infection with a strain of the poliovirus and that most of the time this infection produces no noticeable symptoms—but does produce antibodies that prevent future infection. The younger you are when you're infected, moreover, the better your chances of having a mild reaction and no paralysis. In fact, for most of human history, a large percentage of many populations may have been infected with this virus in early infancy, showed no symptoms, and then developed lifelong immunity. Only occasionally did infection result in any symptoms, which accounts for the fact that lameness following fevers was sporadic. But as the nineteenth century progressed, sanitary reforms in Western countries changed all that. No longer were people living in crowded, unsanitary conditions, and no longer were infants so frequently exposed to the poliovirus. Thus, when a poliovirus did happen to get into the population—perhaps carried by an immune traveler from a less sanitary locale, perhaps encountered by soldiers living in a Third World country where most of the population was immune but the virus was pervasive—epidemics resulted. And these epidemics were serious, because they afflicted children and young adults, who were more susceptible to the severe aftereffects of polio than were infants. Today, of course, most people in developed nations are immune again, thanks to the development of the polio vaccine.

The polio story shows that changing the environment (cleaning up the world) changed poliomyelitis from an endemic disease of infants to an epidemic disease of infants, children, and young adults. With the development of serological testing for antibodies, it became clear that most people living under conditions of crude sanitation developed an immunity to polio in infancy, while people living in "modern," developed nations remained susceptible. Paul explains:

> What happened was that the circulation of polioviruses became more spotty and intermittent as the twentieth century progressed; children arrived at school age and even adolescence without having been exposed or infected, i.e., they remained as susceptibles. Accordingly, they became increasingly vulnerable, and when, inevitably, the virus was introduced after an interval of some years, it spread rapidly through an awaiting susceptible population much as happens with measles. The result was periodic *epidemics* of the disease.[9]

This scenario also suggests that any change in environment—perhaps increased pollution or space travel—can turn what is now accepted as a full-fledged disease into a nameless disease. So, too, can an effective treatment. In recent years, many patients with the ostensibly well-recognized disease syphilis (which is undergoing a resurgence owing to changing socioeconomic factors) have been going from doctor to doctor, diagnosed as having cancers, abscesses, hemorrhoids, hernias, Meniere's disease, multiple sclerosis, and other conditions—all because, since the advent of penicillin, a great many doctors have little experience with this once-prevalent disease.[10]

▲ NAMING: THE SCIENCE UNDERLYING THE PRACTICE

Ultimately, nameless diseases are so difficult for practitioners to name because the medical profession remains uncertain about the exact meaning of the names. This uncertainty involves another aspect of naming, the scientific side. When doctors can't decide *which* name to assign to a patient and what to do about it, that is a problem of medical practice, specifically a problem of diagnosis and treatment. When doctors and researchers can't decide *what* each name involves, however— that is, which specific symptoms, outcomes, and rates of occurrence to include under a generalized name—we are no longer in the realm of medical practice but in that of medical science. And while this scientific side of naming remains inchoate, it is even more difficult to get the patient properly "named." These two aspects of naming, the scientific and the practical, are inextricably connected, for if the medical scientists don't get the names right in the first place, we can't expect practitioners to assign these names correctly to individual patients.

Consider diabetes mellitus ("diabetes"), for example, a condition that most people assume is a disease. Today, however, the American Diabetes Association has divided this "disease" into two types: type I and type II. Each type is also called a "disease." Although all patients with any type of diabetes mellitus, by definition, have problems regulating blood sugar levels, the root of these problems may be so different that doctors have decided to consider type I and type II diabetes different diseases. Patients with type I disease usually develop diabetes before age twenty-five and must take the hormone insulin on a regular basis to control their blood sugar levels. These people are normally of average weight. In contrast, type II disease strikes an entirely different sort of person and in an entirely different sort of way. Patients with type II diabetes—which tends to run in families—are often overweight and usually develop diabetes as adults. With proper diet, these patients may be able to live without insulin injections. Furthermore, pathologists can identify large differences in blood and tissue between these patients and those with type I disease; in fact, it now looks as if each type of diabetes has a different set of causes.

All of this raises the question of whether medical scientists use the term "diabetes" to describe one disease or to include two distinct diseases. Complicating matters further, recent experience suggests that there may be still more "types" of diabetes. For example, there is gestational diabetes, which occurs in pregnant women who have never shown signs of diabetes before, and diabetes due to abnormalities in the insulin molecules themselves (in contrast, insulin molecules in type I and type II diabetes have normal molecular structure; problems come either from impaired secretion or from impaired use of this normal insulin). Are these all different forms of the same "disease," or are they four different diseases? Indeed, are they diseases at all or just symptoms of some larger phenomenon we don't know about yet? And does it matter?

It does matter, very much. If scientists don't know what they mean by a disease name, we can hardly expect a practitioner to diagnose a patient properly. Nor can we expect a practitioner to treat the patient appropriately. If it's "a cold," doctors prescribe bed rest; if it's "a streptococcal infection," they prescribe penicillin. Likewise, if it's "type I diabetes," they prescribe insulin; if it's "type II," they may not—but they'll probably suggest a low-calorie diet and an exercise regimen.

Puerperal mental illness provides an even clearer example of a disease with a problematic definition. Consider the new mother, discussed above, who was diagnosed as having "manic depression" rather than "postpartum [puerperal] depression." Her psychiatrist might have done so because he's a poor diagnostician or because he hasn't kept up on the literature of new diseases or simply because he knows the literature but hasn't found it convincing. Whatever the reason, the failure to recognize or accept "postpartum depression" as a legitimate diagnostic category translates into what some doctors would consider a problem of medical practice. These doctors, however, who believe that postpartum depression is a unique disease, would argue that such a decision of medical practice stems ultimately from a problem of medical science: they'd say that the psychiatrist's decision had less to do with misdiagnosis than with the fact that the medical science he studied didn't recognize postpartum depression as a distinct disease. Trained as he has been, this psychiatrist might be expected to prescribe certain drugs for his patient's "manic depression," the same drugs he would give anyone with this disease, whether or not she had just had a baby. Doctors who believe that postpartum depression is a unique disease would add that if this woman is breast-feeding, some of these drugs—such as lithium—might be excreted with the milk and impair the baby's development then or in later life.[11] On the other hand, if the psychiatrist should decide to commit the woman to a mental hospital and separate her from her infant, the bond between mother and child would obviously suffer.

But consider what might have happened if this practitioner had recognized puerperal mental illness. Chances are good that he would have diagnosed "postpartum depression," rather than "manic depression," and would have made entirely different decisions about care. Understanding that postpartum mental illness is often temporary, he may have decided that drugs like lithium were unnecessary. He might also have vetoed a mental hospital, choosing to hospitalize mother and infant together where they could be monitored. Clearly the medical science underlying a specific diagnosis makes a big difference for the baby's physical and emotional health.

It makes a big difference for the mother as well. In fact, if a woman is not classified as medically ill at all—whether because of a doctor's ignorance of puerperal mental illness or because of medicine's ignorance of puerperal mental illness—she might not only be misled, but might be convicted of a crime! Dr. James Alexander Hamilton has related a truly moving example of the importance of the medical science underlying medical practice, one I think worth repeating. He tells of a woman who gave birth to a baby boy back in the 1840s—a decade in which many doctors still recognized postpartum mental illness as a distinct disease.[12] Word spread through the neighborhood that the new mother wasn't feeling well, and nine days later the local doctor—no fancy specialist—diagnosed her as having a form of puerperal mental illness. Familiar with the condition, he ordered that the mother and baby be separated; he also advised that the woman's friends and neighbors watch over her constantly. A few days later, unfortunately, the friends were all busy, and the woman's thirteen-year-old daughter took charge. When her mother ordered her to bring in the baby, the child had to obey; she also had to obey some time later when her mother asked for a razor so she could remove a callus from her hand. Predictably, this woman used the razor to kill her baby. A trial took place soon thereafter, and the jury decided within a few minutes that this woman was "not guilty by reason of insanity." Three months after the death of the baby, the case had been settled.

However, things turned out quite differently for a California woman who gave birth to a baby boy in 1976. According to Hamilton, about ten days after the delivery, the woman decided something was wrong: she thought that the child made a strange animal cry and that her "head was flying." But no one would believe there was a problem—not her mother, her minister, her pediatrician, not even the orthopedic surgeon who set the child's bone after the new mother had broken it.

Within a few months, this woman had crushed and beaten her baby to death and shot herself in the abdomen. The legal proceedings were time-consuming and complex, costing more than seven years in legal action, trials, prison time, and probation. Moreover, while out on bail, the woman became pregnant again, and she was left by her husband at one point in the trial process.[13]

As Hamilton writes, "The 1847 case was handled with medical wisdom and sophistication. Death followed an accidental failure of a control measure. The case was completed three months after the incident."[14] Contrast this with the unnecessary pain and suffering that occurred more than a hundred years later, when nobody recognized puerperal psychosis as a disease. Clearly, if medical science doesn't recognize a disease, the consequences can be severe for the person suffering from it.

The lack of a clear definition also has grave implications for medical research. Inadequate definition all too frequently results in research errors, errors that ultimately affect patient care. Just think, for instance, about the statisticians who compile records of disease rates: if two different statisticians define cancer in two different ways, it is quite clear that the cancer rates they report are going to differ. Similarly, the statistician who, say, considers postpartum depression as identical to general depression will draw different conclusions than the statistician who separates the two types of depression. These sorts of occurrences have repercussions on the way doctors practice medicine and on how they decide what issues are important and what treatments work.

Although doctors recognize, for example, that there are many forms of epilepsy—including petit mal seizures and partial seizures—many researchers unfortunately have lumped together patients with many different types of epilepsy when testing new drugs and have possibly concluded—erroneously—that certain drugs are useless.[15] A drug that works for petit mal epilepsy may have no effect on partial seizures, but the investigator who studies patients with both forms of epilepsy may erroneously conclude that the drug is useless for any form of epilepsy; the effect on patients with petit mal epilepsy will be statistically washed out by the lack of effect on patients with partial seizures. The same types of problems result every day from assigning the same name to conditions that may require differentiation—conditions such as endometriosis and adenomyosis, dyslexia and other learning disabilities, PMS and various personality disorders, puerperal psychosis and other mental illnesses, various types of anemia, and various forms of cancer.[16] And if the name isn't right in the lab, we can be sure that the name won't be right in the doctor's office either—not to mention the treatment.

▲ ELLIE'S INTERSTITIAL CYSTITIS

It isn't all that surprising that Ellie's doctor mistook her complaint for cystitis and then, when the tests proved him wrong, decided that there was nothing physically wrong with her. Although interstitial cystitis affects thousands of women, few people knew about it until recently. In the past few years researchers and nonmedical support groups have begun meeting formally to discuss the problem and/or to allow sufferers to share experiences, but it takes a long time for new knowledge to filter down to most working doctors: laboratory findings take years to merit publication in specialty journals and even more time to find a place in the medical texts. Even after new knowledge makes it into print, working doctors are bombarded with so many new studies every day that they can't be expected to absorb every obscure detail. Eventually, even the most oblivious doctor will hear about truly important changes in his field, but in some cases this can take decades. Consequently, for many practicing physicians, interstitial cystitis does not exist.

Doctors still don't know the cause (or causes) of this disease, but they do know that somehow the tissue between the lining and muscular wall of the bladder becomes damaged.[17] The degenerated and scarred tissue produces pain around the bladder and the abdomen; it also leads to the extremely frequent urination that Ellie was experiencing. To diagnose interstitial cystitis properly, a doctor must insert a small viewing instrument into the bladder through the urethra to see if there are any characteristic signs of the disease—such as tiny areas of bleeding all over the bladder wall.

If Ellie's doctor had known about interstitial cystitis, he might have been able to offer her some relief. Although there is still no total cure, dilating the bladder seems to help some women, and an anti-inflammatory drug, DMSO (dimethyl sulfoxide), seems to provide temporary relief when instilled directly into the bladder. Meanwhile, the Federal Drug Administration is testing several other promising drugs.

Interstitial cystitis is a nameless disease simply because many doctors still don't know about it and because its symptoms make it look like some better-known diseases. Presumably, this disease will in time be generally recognized and women won't have to run around seeing doctor after doctor, afraid that no one will ever understand what they are going through. They will no longer be called hypochondriacs—and, therefore, will no longer be pushed, like other victims of nameless diseases, into *becoming* hypochondriacs, obsessed with their illness because no one will pay attention to them. One woman, luckier than Ellie, eventually found some support and lived to tell about it on a national talk show. After bouts with four different doctors, she at last found one who knew something about interstitial cystitis and put her in touch with other women with the same complaint. For Ellie, however, this is all irrelevant. She is too busy looking up the name of a good psychiatrist.

▲ TOMMY'S DYSLEXIA

Dyslexia is another condition that is undergoing an identity crisis. Not everyone sees it this way, though; in fact, to hear some people talk, you would think that we already know an awful lot about dyslexia (or specific language disability). According to the Orton Dyslexia Society, this condition affects one-tenth or more of the U.S. population. These people learn to read, write, and spell with much more difficulty than would be expected given their other abilities and opportunities. Dyslexia, the society tells us, literally means a poor or inadequate (*dys*) learning or mastery of verbal language (*lexia*).[18] Persons with dyslexia usually have average intelligence, vision, hearing, motor control, and physical development as well as typical home, school, and emotional lives (except for possible reactions to the frustration of their language difficulties). People with dyslexia may even have great gifts in areas that don't involve language, as noted in Chapter 1. What distinguishes these people, though, are certain behaviors and mannerisms, including the following:

Learning to speak later than most children.

Errors in letter-naming and writing.

Difficulty in learning and remembering printed words.

Impaired reading and writing comprehension.

Reversal of letters or sequences of letters when read or written: for example, *b–d; was–saw; quite–quiet.* (One cartoon shown at an Orton Dyslexia Society meeting depicted a person with dyslexia campaigning for contributions to support dyslexia research. His sign read: "Help Daily Sex.")

Cramped or illegible handwriting as well as a slow rate of writing.

Difficulty in finding the "right" word when speaking— "that thing you use to write with" instead of "pen"; "yesterday" instead of "tomorrow." His syllables and words can come out in the wrong order: "basgetti and cheese" or "please up hurry."

Similar problems among these people's relatives.

This specific kind of language disability may have existed for a long time, but "dyslexia" was unknown until the late nineteenth century. One explanation for this is that literate societies are a fairly recent phenomenon; for most of human existence, problems with language were neither obvious nor relevant. Even when literacy started to matter, the handicaps of dyslexia usually had only a minimal impact, particularly if they were accompanied by superior abilities in other areas. Indeed, a gene for dyslexia might have been an adaptation that allowed society to produce many different individuals with different talents.

Early in this century, however, a scattering of psychologists and educators began to notice that language disabilities had a subtle but worrisome impact on human learning, working, and emotional life. In the 1930s, the work of the neurologist Samuel Torrey Orton, director of the Green County Medical Clinic in Ohio, made tremendous strides toward the understanding and educational management of language development. Orton made these studies his life's work, and eventually the Orton Dyslexia Society was named after him.[19]

In recent years, members of the Orton Dyslexia Society, as well as other dyslexia authorities, have noted that people with dyslexia often share certain traits in addition to their language problems. Dyslexic children may be underachievers who behave impulsively in school, or they may be overly meticulous. They may be ambidextrous, disorganized, hyperactive, confused about directions in space or time (right and left, up and down, yesterday and tomorrow), and mathematically handicapped (or gifted!). But, again, a person doesn't need to have any of these traits to be called "dyslexic": anyone who has trouble with language despite an adequate IQ and normal environment may have dyslexia.

This definition seems simple enough and, indeed, quite solid. Closer scrutiny, however, shows why there is so much confusion about the meaning of the term "dyslexia." To understand why, just ask yourself what "trouble with language," "adequate IQ," and "normal environment" mean exactly. A little thought reveals how loose these terms actually are; they are not bounded by quantitative limits or measurable with laboratory tests. Deciding whether someone has grown up in a "normal environment," for example, requires a subjective judgment about what is "normal."

Consequently, many people are skeptical about whether the term "dyslexia" really refers to one specific condition or whether one word is being used to describe several heterogeneous learning problems. Many doctors and psychologists, for example, suspect that dyslexia is not a "real" disease in itself but merely a shorthand term for a symptom (language troubles) that can accompany many diseases. They ignore the language problems per se and, depending on what other traits their patient may have, diagnose the root of the problem as "minimal brain damage," "attention deficit disorder," "clumsy child syndrome," "hyperactivity," "visual motor perceptual lag," "organic brain disease," "learning disorder," or "minimal cerebral palsy." Thus, what we originally thought was a clearly defined term meaning "language problem" suddenly has more than half a dozen possible names.

Of course, everyone could be right. It is possible, after all, that the simple name "dyslexic" actually comprehends several different groups of people, some of whom merely have language troubles with no other symptoms while others have language troubles owing to other diseases. Not everyone who has trouble learning to read, after all, necessarily has the same problem: some may have a mild dysfunction in their brains; some may have certain brain cells that work differently (not worse) than most people's; some may have subtle emotional problems; some may have foreign chemicals that cause their neural connections to go haywire; and others may simply be lazy.

The real confusion, though, comes from people who do not recognize this possible heterogeneity. Some authorities when pressed will acknowledge that, yes, the term "dyslexia" may actually refer to several different categories of language difficulty. But in everyday practice they assume that dyslexia is dyslexia is dyslexia. Worse still, after a while laxness leads them to start using the various names for language troubles interchangeably. In 1985, for example, an article in the Brown University alumni magazine stated that "attention deficit syndrome" is a characteristic of dyslexia—not a separate condition of only some people with dyslexia. Even leading authorities will use terms like "hyperactivity" and "dyslexia" as though they were synonymous, as if everyone with hyperactivity had dyslexia and vice versa. Speakers at scientific symposiums have described studies of "dyslexic" children and then applied conclusions to all children with "learning disabilities." It's no wonder, then, that when one mother notices that Tommy, the boy next door—whose grades are poor just like her own son's—has been labeled dyslexic, she decides that her seven-year-old son has dyslexia, too. It sounds a lot better than "minimally brain-damaged" or "irresponsible."

On the other hand, how can Tommy's mother prove that her otherwise normal son is having trouble reading because of dyslexia when teachers theorize that the problem is much simpler: the child would rather watch television than read Dick and Jane? Skeptics pose this question as they watch "dyslexia" bandied about by anyone and everyone, applied to many different children as a euphemistic catchall term for brain damage, retardation, laziness, or behavior problems. Combined with ignorance of dyslexia's symptoms, this skepticism also explains why Tommy was kept back in school so long.

▲ GAIL'S PREMENSTRUAL SYNDROME

Finally, let's look at PMS, one of the better-known nameless diseases. It's so well known, in fact, that it's quickly leaving the "nameless" stage: many people clearly believe that PMS is a full-fledged medical entity. Just think of all the PMS clinics springing up across the United States (the first one opened in Boston in 1981), all the talk shows debating whether women with PMS should be acquitted of crimes, and all the newspapers regularly reporting new PMS cures. Furthermore, all you have to do is go into your local bookshop, and you'll spot three or four colorful paperbacks promising to explain your PMS to you. PMS is so "in," in fact, that it's even made the *Wall Street Journal*.[20]

But, as Gail's case indicates, publicity does not mean that this condition has achieved universal recognition as a legitimate disease. Just because there is a book "on" something, after all, doesn't mean that something exists; it is equally possible that women find it useful to be-lieve in PMS, and there's a lot of money to be made on books catering to this belief. There are a lot of books on ghosts, too, but that is no guaran-tee that ghosts exist. At any rate, this is what many people are still argu-ing, and they point out quite correctly that, so far, no one has shown that PMS is a unique physical condition provoked by something spe-cific like a bacterium or a hormonal imbalance or characterized by distinct behavior patterns. This kind of thinking led the American Psy-chiatric Association in July 1986 to bar PMS from its list of officially rec-ognized mental disorders.[21]

But none of this means that something very unpleasant isn't happening to a lot of women and that something shouldn't be done about it. It is quite true that the scientific community still hasn't agreed upon an exact definition of PMS—but that doesn't mean that the people who use the term aren't referring to a very clear problem. First de-scribed in 1931 by Dr. Robert Frank, this problem was originally known as "premenstrual tension." In 1954, however, Dr. Katharina Dalton (considered by many to be the founder of the PMS field) and Raymond Greene proposed changing "tension" to "syndrome"—since there are many other aspects of the condition beside tension.[22]

Today the difference between "premenstrual syndrome" and "premenstrual tension" is rather unclear: both terms are used, some-times interchangeably, to describe any of hundreds of symptoms that occur up to fifteen days before and stop by the end of the first day of menstruation. For some women improved diet, regular exercise, and/or vitamin supplements relieve mild to moderate symptoms; for others, clinics and doctors are trying more drastic measures, not al-ways successfully.

Once a month, women who have this syndrome, popularly known as "PMS," develop one or more of about a hundred different symptoms, including bloating, nausea, headaches, sleep disorders, moodiness, depression, fatigue, anxiety, vomiting, sweating, acne, weight gain, joint swelling, and nervousness. These are just examples of the symptoms: what characterizes PMS is not the particular symp-tom(s) but rather its (or their) recurrence every month in the five to fifteen days before the menstrual period begins.[23] To some extent, al-most all women experience some version of PMS. After all, hormonal levels have emotional as well as physical influences—the hormone tes-tosterone can control sexual desire and hair growth, for example—and it only makes sense that the hormone levels characteristic of the pre-menstrual phase would produce unique effects. Not surprisingly, then, the American Council for Science and Health estimated in 1985 that the majority—maybe even 90 percent—of all women experience some physical or psychological changes during the week before menstruation.

It is only when this perhaps normal reaction to shifting hormonal levels becomes disabling that PMS requires medical attention. And for 20 to 40 percent of women, symptoms in the days before menstruation are indeed severe enough to interfere with normal activities. Some women develop severe headaches and nausea; others feel violent impulses that impel them to strike out randomly (for example, one woman from Saskatoon, Saskatchewan, told her doctor that when she felt that way she got into her car and went looking for someone to hit).

Not everyone would agree, however, that PMS is merely an overreaction to normal conditions. Other researchers have suggested that the syndrome is caused by abnormally low hormone levels, disturbed hormonal regulation or balance, low blood sugar, water retention, vitamin deficiencies, and, of course, psychological problems. Others suggest that more than one of these factors may be involved.

Of course, it's also possible that what we are calling PMS is not one condition with one explanation, but several separate conditions. From this perspective, "PMS" is a generic term like the "flu," rather than a specific term like "German measles." When we have the "flu" we know our muscles ache just like Uncle Jack's did when he had the "flu." But Uncle Jack had the Hong Kong flu, a different condition from our swine flu, despite the common name and common symptom. Similarly, it may turn out that a woman who experiences bloating and nausea premenstrually may actually have an entirely different kind of condition than one who experiences headaches and anxiety. In other words, even though the timing and some of the symptoms may be similar, there may be several forms of PMS—each with a different explanation and overall pattern of symptoms. If this were true, then Gail's "PMS" might be related to low hormone levels while her friend Jackie's "PMS" might be related to a vitamin deficiency. So far, though, no one has been able to divide PMS into consistent types.

Of course, just because PMS has different forms doesn't necessarily preclude it from being a distinct disease. Rheumatic fever, after all, is a disease that consists of five diverse major manifestations (including arthritis, a painless rash, and involuntary jerky movements) that can appear alone or in various combinations. According to Glenn O. Bair, a Topeka, Kansas, clinician, PMS may turn out to be a similar type of disease. "It was very difficult over the decades to describe all of the symptoms of rheumatic fever and to make an appropriate diagnosis," he told me. "Finally, however, when we agreed upon the Jones criteria [the patient has to have at least two major or one major and two minor manifestations], a diagnosis of probable rheumatic fever in children can be made. Perhaps PMS will be identified in similar fashion."

Still, other people insist, as some do with respect to dyslexia, that PMS is not a syndrome or disease at all, but just a symptom of some larger problem or problems. Here PMS would be comparable to something like insomnia—a problem that can be a symptom with many causes: anxiety, depression, breathing difficulties, stress, and so on. If this is true, then doctors who want to treat PMS should be looking for the disease underlying it.

What is the truth? We don't know yet. We can theorize all we want and believe what makes us happiest, but until the scientific evidence becomes available, we'll just have to go on and decide how to think about a lot of uncomfortable women—and doctors will have to decide how to treat them.

And that is where the difficulties begin. Because there is no clear definition of PMS, and because many doctors doubt that it is a "real" disease, misdiagnosis is common—as it is for interstitial cystitis and dyslexia and all the other nameless diseases. In part this is so because the symptoms of PMS can resemble those in many other conditions, including dysmenorrhea, epilepsy, endometriosis, pelvic inflammatory disease, a pituitary tumor, an underactive thyroid gland, as well as psychiatric conditions such as manic-depressive disorder and chronic depression. In fact, some doctors diagnose "PMS" only if they have ruled out every other possibility; for them, the term has no meaning in itself except that no other explanation can be found for the patient's symptoms.[24] Besides ignoring the real problem, a false diagnosis can mean inappropriate medications—most of which are worthless, counterproductive, or even dangerous.[25]

Complicating the situation, then, is the fact that other conditions such as an underactive thyroid gland, depression, or schizophrenia often produce symptoms that are also associated with PMS.[26] In fact, some studies suggest that many or even most women with severe premenstrual depression (but without other symptoms of PMS) may have some sort of psychiatric illness. Doctors familiar with these studies may assume that any woman who comes in with the symptoms of PMS is "really" a psychiatric or thyroid case in disguise; they don't realize that she just might simply have PMS or might have PMS in addition to another disease. Furthermore, once they rule out all other diseases, they might tell her, as Gail's doctors did, that there is nothing wrong that a little self-discipline wouldn't cure.

▲ LOOKING FOR A MARKER

At this point it might seem that the scientific and medical communities are full of shortsighted, muddleheaded people, completely oblivious to a disease your next-door neighbor could tell them about. But, to be fair, there are roadblocks to perfect medical knowledge. As we saw with interstitial cystitis, for example, it takes years for new medical knowledge to be verified experimentally and even more years for it to reach the average practitioner; despite valiant effort, no doctor can instantaneously absorb the thousands of studies published every month.

Matters are even more complicated for doctors grappling with dyslexia and PMS. Like many other psychological or behavioral diseases, these conditions are hard to define with the rigor of something like rubella (German measles) or tuberculosis. A disease seems more legitimate if it has an associated biological marker—some easy-to-measure physical or biochemical event that appears in all cases of the disease. In tuberculosis, the biological marker is the *Mycobacterium tuberculosis,* the bacterium found in the blood of people with tuberculosis. If you show enough of the right symptoms and signs (a sign is a clue to disease that results from a doctor's examination)—and you have this biological marker—then doctors can confidently diagnose tuberculosis. In contrast, many of today's nameless diseases have emotional or behavioral components that make it difficult to squeeze them into modern definitions of disease given doctors' marked preference for biological and physical explanations.

Emotional symptoms have no clear beginning, middle, and end. As Ann Nazzaro and Donald Lombard explain in their book on PMS, although emotional symptoms have an underlying biological explanation, emotional symptoms "do not seem scientifically real because they cannot be measured, they cannot be prodded and tested, and they can be difficult to separate from specific circumstances."[27] In other words, it is harder to define and explain a vague feeling of anxiety, pegging it to a specific set of circumstances, than it is to say that a rash resulted from a reaction to the measles virus.

Not surprisingly, then, psychiatric diseases, which often involve emotions and behaviors not yet (and perhaps never to be) linked with some specific physical event, are notorious for their shifting defini- tions.[28] Thus, the decision to recategorize PMS was hardly unique. Psy- chiatrists are constantly debating about where to draw the boundaries between different mental diseases, how to determine the reliability and validity of their diagnoses, and even whether certain behaviors can be called mental diseases at all. The psychiatric profession's gradual ac- ceptance of alcoholism as a disease and the American Psychiatric Asso- ciation's decree in late 1973 that most forms of homosexuality are not diseases are only some of the best-publicized instances of the sort of reclassification that goes on constantly.

One reason for these frequent changes may be the relative new- ness of the field of psychiatry. In fact, as late as the mid-nineteenth cen- tury, many doctors regarded "insanity" in general as the one and only mental disease; there were no formal divisions into categories such as "paranoid schizophrenia" or "obsessive-compulsive disorder."[29] Today, psychiatric researchers have made significant strides toward formally distinguishing many kinds of mental illness and improving the relia- bility and validity of their diagnoses, but there is still significant overlap and reliance on subjective, individual judgment. Another explanation for the frequent changes may be the social and political forces that can stigmatize psychiatric patients. At times, people labeled as having a mental disease want to be defined out of the disease category and re- garded as psychologically "normal."

But, again, the lack of a biological marker remains the funda- mental explanation for the frequently shifting names and categories of mental diseases. As we will see later, having a biological marker is not a prerequisite for a condition to be identifiable as a unique disease; many quite legitimate diseases, both medical and psychiatric, can be diagnosed from characteristic symptoms or histories.[30] It certainly makes things easier, however, when a reading from a lab test or a mark on an X-ray can prove once and for all that this disease is different from all other conditions. PMS would certainly be easier to peg if someone could show a biological trait unique to all women with certain vague emotional and behavioral symptoms. So would conditions like "lone- liness" and "stress" that somehow account for unhappiness and that may predispose people to sniffles, heart attacks, and even certain kinds of cancer. At the same time, an "objective" physical marker would make it much harder to confuse the vague somatic complaints (e.g., fatigue, nausea, vomiting, weakness, paralysis, headache, abdominal pain, or dysmenorrhea) attributable to nameless diseases with psychiatric conditions such as "hysteria" and "hypochondria."

Behavioral diseases such as dyslexia are similarly problematic. People with dyslexia by definition have no obvious physical defects, but at a microscopic level something in the brain may not be working the way it does for most people.[31] If we knew that there is a distinct problem with the cells of a dyslexic brain—that they are abnormal in form or slack in function—then it would be easy to examine a child and say, "Oh, yes, he definitely has dyslexia. He's not faking or lazy or emotionally disturbed. It's just that a few of his brain cells have an unusual configuration."

Almost since dyslexia was first described, investigators have been trying to find out what that unusual configuration might be, and today the Orton Dyslexia Society sponsors a "brain bank" and CAT scans to determine the characteristics of dyslexic brains. For all the theories proposed over the years, though, concrete proof remains extremely elusive.

Admittedly, some findings are intriguing. One group of researchers, for example, looked at the brain cells from four different men who had had dyslexia and described their characteristics; the results suggest strongly that at least some dyslexia may occur when certain brain cells develop abnormally.[32] Another researcher examined the brains of normal boys and of boys with dyslexia and found electrical differences in the regions involved in speech and reading,[33] while still others have found that metabolic activity may differ in certain regions of the dyslexic brain.[34] There is even some evidence that dyslexia may at times be associated with a chromosomal defect; eventually, researchers hope to know whether this defect causes some specific physical or biochemical abnormality.[35]

Similarly intriguing findings are also beginning to appear with respect to chronic fatigue immune dysfunction syndrome, another nameless disease. Although links to specific viruses or immune-system disorders have thus far been discredited, there is some evidence of anomalies in the electrical activity of the brain associated with CFIDS—namely, anomalies in the temporal lobes, which are areas that help regulate emotions and survival responses. There is also some evidence that people with CFIDS have trouble encoding new memories and that immune-system modulators and antiviral agents can restore the temporal lobes to normal function.[36] Again, though, since most of these investigations have involved only a handful of patients, the search for a physical or biochemical marker must continue, and people with language disability as well as those with inexplicable chronic fatigue and flulike symptoms must still battle for their "name."

The lack of a biological marker does not just hinder definition; it also makes people doubt that the illness exists at all, as we have already seen in such nameless diseases as PMS and dyslexia. The dominant American society generally dismisses as "imaginary" anything it can't explain in terms of physical cause. Consider a common reaction to certain illnesses reported among a diverse group of Hispanics in the U.S. Southwest, for example.[37] These people have illnesses that don't "exist" insofar as mainstream Western medicine is concerned; medical students don't learn about them, patients don't complain of them, and the treatments that work for these Hispanic Americans don't make sense according to current medical theory.

And yet, for the group of Hispanics surveyed, these are very real and very understandable diseases. In one of them—known as *susto,* or "fright sickness"—victims experience depression, insomnia, irritability, nervousness, and diarrhea after any startling event. Weak teas can calm mild cases, but a ritual cleansing (*barrida*) in which objects are brushed over the body to the chant of prayers may be necessary as well. In another disease, called *empacho,* which mainly afflicts children, the intestines seem to be blocked, and the result is a bloated stomach, constipation, indigestion, diarrhea, vomiting, and lethargy; to treat *empacho,* healers administer herbal teas and give massages. And finally, infants with *caída de mollera* have a depressed soft spot on their heads and may become irritable, weepy, dehydrated, and feverish. The Hispanics surveyed believe this disease may be caused by pulling the baby away from the breast or bottle too quickly, and they commonly treat it by pushing up on the baby's palate, holding the child upside down, and hitting the heels.

How can we explain these diseases, which almost no one has heard of in Des Moines, Iowa, but which are known to nearly every ten-year-old in certain Hispanic villages of the U.S. Southwest? Our gut reaction might be that the particular Hispanics surveyed are ignorant and primitive and that these "diseases" are the misguided machinations of their untrained minds. They believe in *susto* like they believe in the tree god; they simply can't think straight, and they make things up that make them feel better. But there are several other explanations that put these "diseases" in a more sympathetic light. For one thing, there could be a local germ that lives only in the hot, dry regions of the Southwest and thrives among the Hispanics there because of some peculiar hygienic practice or genetic quirk. Or perhaps a contaminated local well is spreading the germs of *susto, empacho,* and *caída de mollera.* It's also possible that these diseases are just other names for conditions we already know; *caída de mollera,* for example, might be a form of colic.

The most likely explanation, however, is that this particular group of Hispanics simply sees the world differently than we do. They are not necessarily less sophisticated or realistic; they simply see different events as worthy of attention, so that what we think of as normal they think of as disease. For example, imagine meeting a woman who has just seen her child jump from a tree and break a leg. We might react by saying, "She's naturally a bit upset, but the child's all taped up now and she'll get over it." But a Hispanic observer might notice what we don't—that the woman becomes depressed and has trouble sleeping. This observer might then link these new developments with the recent shock and call it *susto.* Once that is established, it's hardly surprising that the calming influence of a friend offering tea or a massage or even the passage of time would help relieve the symptoms.

From this perspective, what originally seemed bizarre becomes understandable: *susto* is a distinct condition with a known cause (shock), specific symptoms (insomnia, depression, etc.), and an effective treatment (teas and massage). That's a lot better than we can say for a much less bizarre disease known as the common cold.

That a particular group of Hispanics might see things as significant that we don't seems like a very simple and probable explanation for *susto, empacho,* and *caída de mollera.* And yet, what is most interesting here is that even the very enlightened among us who would never call these Hispanics "crazy" or "primitive" seem never to have thought of this simple explanation. Rather, proponents of these diseases argue that *susto, empacho,* and *caída de mollera* may well be linked to biological conditions recognized in mainstream medicine; they believe that connecting these behavioral symptoms with some well-known physical explanation is the only way to prove that they are not imaginary.[38] By never considering that these diseases might be real from a different point of view, they imply that any complaint that doesn't have a recognized biological marker must be "all in the mind." This is the same attitude that people with nameless diseases face every day.

There's a catch here, of course. Before you can look for a biological marker, you have to believe that the disease actually exists as a unique entity. There is no point in searching for a biological marker for an "I-don't-want-to-practice-the-piano syndrome" if you think this is just a ploy exhibited by a diverse group of children for a variety of reasons. This situation traps many nameless diseases into a vicious circle: without a biological marker, nameless diseases are considered imaginary; and, since they are considered to be imaginary, no one will look for a biological marker.

CHAPTER 3

▲

The Difficulty of Naming Diseases

▲ IS A BROKEN ANKLE A DISEASE?

A rose may be a rose may be a rose, but a cold's not a cold. Different people "have colds" in different ways: Jenny sneezes and Johnny coughs; Tammy aches for days and Tommy muddles through school despite the sniffles. Even if several people all have a disease with the same name, no two patients have identical experiences. Yet, doctors lump certain experiences together as examples of specific diseases. What is it that makes doctors know what to lump with what? How do they know that while Jenny sneezes and Johnny coughs, both have a "cold"?

First, let's consider Johnny. A few days ago, he felt a slightly sore itchiness in his throat, and yesterday he started to cough to relieve the tickle. Today he is hacking loudly every few minutes, and he feels so drained that his mother lets him stay home from school. She phones the pediatrician, who tells her that Johnny probably "has a cold" and who asks her to take the boy's temperature. When she reports that Johnny has no fever, the doctor recommends plenty of rest and orange juice.

Now consider Jenny. Up until yesterday she'd felt perfectly fine, if a little tired. She woke up sneezing yesterday morning, however, and by four o'clock that afternoon she had to keep a box of tissues at her side to combat the drippiness. At six, she took her temperature and found she had a fever of 101 degrees. She took two aspirin, and by morning her temperature was normal. In fact, despite some sniffles, she felt well enough to go to work. She tells her coworkers to keep their distance, however, because she has a "cold."

Jenny's experience is different from Johnny's, but they have certain things in common, and both call their conditions "colds." What about Jenny's experience tells her that she has a cold, rather than influenza, or rather than a random combination of symptoms or several different diseases? And what about Johnny's experience tells him that he, too, is suffering from this one thing, this "cold"?

When doctors make a diagnosis, they are doing a kind of "fitting," deciding if there is one specific aspect—or many aspects—of a patient's experience (e.g., obvious symptoms, abnormal laboratory results, history of medical problems) that acts as a "clincher," aspects that say "this is a cold rather than a flu." A major issue in deciding how to name a patient's disease, then, is determining which specific aspects of an individual's experience are the clinchers, the ones that count in the fitting; which specific aspect of a disease defines it as a specific entity separate from other diseases. Of course, each practicing physician doesn't have to determine these clinchers for each individual patient; that determination is made by medical scientists who define or name the disease in the first place, and the role of the practitioner is to recognize this clincher and then decide whether it fits a preexisting category.[1] The question that has to be answered, then, before we know how to tell whether Johnny or Jenny has a cold, is how we know that any two experiences represent a cold.

How simple things would be if a common cause were enough to identify two experiences as the same disease! We could simply say, for example, that "both Frieda and Margaret have fevers, but Frieda has a different disease than Margaret because her fever has a different cause." And, in many cases, such reasoning works very well. In separating typhoid fever from scarlet fever, for example, doctors often rely on their knowledge that one disease is "caused" by *Salmonella typhi* and the other by beta-hemolytic streptococci, and that a test for the microorganism present will clinch the matter.[2]

But there are complications in determining a clincher, even in diseases as well defined as typhoid and scarlet fever. These two diseases differ in many respects besides the causative microorganism—patients with scarlet fever rarely develop the abdominal pain characteristic of typhoid fever, for example—and thus it is not knowing the "cause" alone which tells doctors that the two diseases are different. Nor do we always need to know a cause to distinguish one disease from another. We know that cancer is not the same disease as diabetes, for example, even though the causes of both remain mysterious.

Unfortunately, there are no easy answers—even for the common cold. The first thing that both Johnny and Jenny had to do in realizing that they had "colds" was to decide that they were sick, that they had a "disease." They made this decision before they wondered *which* disease they had. True, for Johnny and Jenny this decision was fairly easy to make: both patients "felt lousy," "not up to snuff," or "couldn't function normally." In many cases, though, deciding what is sick and what is healthy is just as difficult as deciding what specifically is wrong. In fact, most medical philosophers agree that what is called "sick" and what is called "healthy" vary from culture to culture.[3]

No one has any problem calling "measles" a disease, but what about a broken arm, a pierced ear, an allergic fit, or a feeling of despair? What about nearsightedness, alcoholism, or the bound feet of ancient Chinese women? For some people, in some places, at some times, these things might be called "injuries" rather than "diseases," "normal" rather than "abnormal," "imaginary" rather than "actual," or "caused by a demon" rather than "caused by a biochemical imbalance." For other people, in other places, at other times, just the opposite might be true.

When we think of disease, moreover, certain notions pop up, but they're not the same notions for everyone. In fact, try defining "disease." One common-sense definition might be "a physical condition that keeps me from functioning normally." Fine. By this definition, measles would be a disease. So would a cold—or a heart attack. Of course, too, there are many physical conditions that keep us from functioning normally which we probably wouldn't call diseases—say, having too many martinis. And then there's the problem of defining what "functioning normally" means in the first place. Functioning normally for me—or for the entire population? For me at age twenty—or at age seventy? It may be normal—in the sense of "average"—for a ninety-year-old person to be dying of heart failure, but we nevertheless would probably want to call that a disease. Perhaps, then, we mean "functioning normally" compared with an average member of the population. But then a six-month-old who couldn't run the fifty-yard dash in under twenty seconds would be considered to have a disease.

Clearly, then, this simple definition is inadequate. What departs from the ordinary is arbitrary, because what is ordinary or normal is arbitrary. Philosophers have been trying for years to come up with a better definition of "disease" by amending this basic definition or suggesting others, but so far no single definition can encompass what every culture regards as disease. In fact, when Christopher Boorse, a medical sociologist, reviewed the literature that discussed what disease is, he found that there is no consistent definition valid for all conditions. For some philosophers, disease has been what is "bad" or "undesirable" from the patient's point of view; for others, it is a condition that requires a doctor's care. Boorse found that still other philosophers have defined disease as a condition that deviates from statistical normality; as a condition that involves pain, suffering, or discomfort; as a condition that produces disability; as a maladaption to environment; as an imbalance among the body's systems; or as a combination of several of these.[4]

Unfortunately, however, it is easy enough to find exceptions to any combination of these definitions: just pick several conditions that you consider to be diseases, and see whether they can be fit into any consistent scheme. The literature of medical philosophy is full of examples suggesting that a universal definition of disease is impossible. There is no point in belaboring them here; the bottom line is simply that although many obviously painful, undesirable conditions are considered unhealthy everywhere at all times, many conditions can be considered normal and healthy in some circumstances and abnormal and unhealthy in others. This does not mean, however, that we cannot define disease.[5] The key is to remember that what is considered unhealthy or diseased varies from culture to culture.

It is not necessary to plod through philosophy or to travel in distant lands to understand that our notion of disease is relative. Even within one society, connotations of the term "disease" vary from person to person. A good illustration of this variation appears in a study reported in the *British Medical Journal*. The authors found that doctors and laymen use the term "disease" in different ways. For laymen, what was most important in labeling something a disease was a living agent (e.g., a bacterium) or the necessity of a doctor's presence. Doctors, on the other hand, were more likely to think of diseases as physical conditions—such as lead poisoning or an allergic reaction to cats—caused by chemical and physical agents. Many doctors also distinguished between injuries and diseases, injuries being caused by *external* physical agents.[6]

▲ PINNING DOWN JOHNNY'S COLD

We have just seen that different cultures—and various groups within the same culture—answer the question "What is disease?" differently. A second, related question, however, is even more difficult to answer: "What is *a* disease?" In other words, what distinguishes one disease from the next? This is a different question from "What is disease?" because it is possible to be unhealthy (or "diseased") and still not have a specific disease. You can have a headache, for example, or you can sneeze. We call these events "symptoms" of diseases, not "diseases" themselves. They provide clues that help us determine what disease we have, and they certainly cannot be regarded as "healthy," but they themselves are not distinct diseases.

To answer our second question, let's return to the "cold" example. Before we can say how we know Johnny or Jenny "has a cold" (i.e., how we diagnose them), we first have to know what we mean by saying that *anyone* "has a cold" (i.e., how scientists name diseases). More generally, we have to know what it means to call anyone's condition a "disease" before we can understand how to diagnose Johnny or Jenny as having one. Most people would say they know what a disease is, of course. Measles is a disease. Mumps is, too. Each of these is a distinct sickness and has certain characteristics that distinguish it from other sicknesses. It's fairly easy to list many obvious examples. To answer the question "What is a disease?" or "What do we mean when we say that someone has a disease?" then, presumably all we have to do is decide what characteristics are necessary for a condition to constitute its own category known as "a disease."

To help us further, medical tomes describe the distinct symptoms, etiologies, prognoses, and therapies for all the known separate diseases that can befall humankind. Even if we can't cure certain specific diseases—such as cancer or heart disease—and even if we don't know what causes all of these conditions, these books imply that there is a specific, well-defined "thing" we can define, even if we can't cure it.

But is there? Things start getting a little rockier when we leave the textbooks that purport to tell us exactly what a "cold" is and ask instead what made the medical scientists decide that experiences like the ones Johnny and Jenny had both constitute the same disease. Do researchers consider two conditions part of one distinct disease only when they have the same cause, when we know they have both the same cause and the same treatment, or when they have three common symptoms and a common cause? Or does the answer to this question vary from disease to disease, according to whim or to pragmatics? The answer will tell us not only how researchers know what to lump with what as a common cold but also how diagnosticians know that Jenny and Johnny both had a cold. Did some specific symptom, such as sneezing, tip them off? Clearly not, since Johnny coughs—he doesn't sneeze—yet we still say he has a cold. Is it a specific sequence of symptoms—say, sneezing followed by coughing several days later? That's what happened to Jenny, but Johnny coughed for several days and then felt well. Perhaps, then, diagnosing a cold means seeing any of a variety of symptoms, but all with a common "cause." But this is not right either, for what we call the common cold may be "caused" by more than a hundred different viruses.

The basic question, whether in naming diseases or diagnosing patients, is how we know when two conditions are separate diseases. It's easy enough to separate measles and mumps and say that they are distinct diseases, but what about lung cancer and prostate cancer? Both share certain qualities—pain, weakness, a small mass of rapidly dividing cells that may spread to other organs—but do both have a common cause? A common outcome? We really don't know, at least not given current medical knowledge. So, at this point in time, can we say they are the same disease?

As a matter of fact, it's hard to know what we mean when we decide that Johnny—leaving out Jenny altogether—"has a cold." Do we mean that something called a "cold," something with all the characteristics described in the textbook, dropped out of the sky, imbedded itself in Johnny, and then left? Perhaps so—a virus may indeed have dropped out of the sky and infected him—but a virus is not a cold; after all, lots of people are exposed to this virus, but only a few of them actually start sneezing.

Maybe, then, having a cold means being infected with a virus and later developing certain symptoms. This definition seems plausible, but it still leaves open the question of when exactly the disease begins. Did Johnny have the disease the day the virus entered his body—even though he felt fine that day—or did he first have the disease when his throat started hurting? When he started sneezing a few days later, was this part of the same "cold" as the sore throat, or did the cold begin on the day he sneezed? Furthermore, was it the same cold on the day he started sneezing or a different cold as his symptoms changed?

Other questions involve the site of the disease. Is the cold in

Johnny's throat, in his nose, in both? If the latter, is it then appropriate to say that Johnny has a cold, or just that he has a cold in his throat and nose? Maybe the cold is in his whole body. If so, though, why does he feel quite normal everywhere but in his head? Furthermore, if the cold really has a physical location, when did it arrive at that point? Was it in his nose, preparing to take effect, on the days when only his throat hurt? [7]

▲ DISEASE AS PATTERN

Without answering any of these questions, people decide every day that certain conditions constitute certain diseases. In practical terms, we're quite clearly able to answer our original question—"At what point do isolated events 'deserve' to be seen as a distinct pattern and called a specific disease?" Somehow we know, though perhaps unconsciously, exactly when to lump isolated symptoms or other features together and call the whole patient experience a disease. Somehow we know when a sniffle is more than a sniffle and becomes part of a cold. And somehow we know how many symptoms—and which ones— it takes to turn having a virus in your blood to having a disease such as a cold.

The truth remains, however, that we really don't know exactly what we mean when we call something a disease. We know what the textbook says about characteristics of the disease and how to match certain patients and their problems with these characteristics, but the implications of having a disease elude us: we don't know what type of being this disease is, when it arrived, where it resides, or when it leaves. We're not even sure whether this disease is a "thing." We have to make our judgments knowing that there is no neat scheme by which all diseases can be lined up, each aspect comparable on a one-for-one basis. Thus, some diseases are distinguished by changes in the body's appearance, some by distinct dysfunctions in the body, and others by the specific microorganism isolated in patients with the disease. Other diseases are distinguished by biochemical changes, a single telling symptom, or one characteristic result of a laboratory test. Still other diseases are distinguished by some combination of these or other features.

For example, some physicians regard basal-cell carcinoma, a form of skin cancer, as a distinct disease because each patient with this condition shows a characteristic *cellular pattern*. Yet the same physicians regard Down's syndrome as a distinct disease not because of a specific cellular appearance, but because patients with Down's syndrome have a characteristic *genetic status*. Furthermore, doctors regard alcoholism as a distinct disease because all patients with alcoholism share certain *individual habits* (e.g., frequent intoxication, which interferes with socializing and work; marital problems; physical injuries; criminal behavior; and driving under the influence), whereas they regard hypertension as a disease because patients with hypertension, who typically don't feel unwell, show one *characteristic sign* (i.e., high blood pressure, which is synonymous with the name of the disease). There is no one aspect shared by all diseases—neither cause nor symptoms nor prognosis nor treatment—which by its uniqueness distinguishes one set of experiences from the next and assures us that a particular set of experiences represents one distinct disease.

Even such medical tomes as the *Manual of the International Statistical Classification of Diseases, Injuries, and Causes of Death* and the *Merck Manual* use inconsistent criteria for labeling an affliction as a distinct disease. Although these manuals, as well as the standard textbooks of medicine, appear to be logically divided exactly on such lines, it turns out that some of the headings refer to "diseases," while others refer to "syndromes" or "disorders" or simply "conditions." Few authors (with the notable exception of research psychiatrists) even attempt to define these terms; in fact, they often use them interchangeably. And even when implicit schemes exist, they vary from author to author. As we'll see throughout this book, some people use "disease" to mean a group of different syndromes; others use "syndrome" to mean a group of different diseases. Furthermore, some people reserve the term "disease" for those conditions which have a known etiology; others use it for any commonly associated group of symptoms, even when the cause is unknown or when there are several different causes.

Perhaps the most reasonable way to distinguish one disease from the next is to view each disease as a unique combination or *pattern*—according to current knowledge and theory—of certain interconnected features such as physical abnormalities, symptoms, patient demographics, timing, prospects for recovery, and/or causal factors. How these features are connected may not be known, but there is the hypothetical assumption that they are not randomly associated and that they have some sort of inner, coherent relationship. Besides having certain anatomical abnormalities, for example, a woman with endometriosis also notices certain symptoms, responds to certain treatments, and falls into certain age and sex categories; it is this specific combination of related factors, rather than any one factor alone, which defines her disease.

Even seeing each disease as a distinct pattern has its problems, however, since what constitutes a legitimate pattern also varies from culture to culture and from disease to disease. In the early nineteenth century, for example, many disease patterns often had nothing at all to do with what caused the disease or with the sex or age of the typical patient. Of course, certain diseases of that time—including some specific contagious diseases such as tetanus—resembled our patterns today. Tetanus then involved a cause (a wound), symptoms (involuntary contraction of muscles), and treatment (cleaning the wound, administering opium and tobacco, and warm baths). Even though some of the specific elements in the pattern differed from our description of tetanus today, the nature of the elements was similar. Quite frequently, though, doctors meant something very different when they spoke of "a disease." In fact, the term often seemed to carry several meanings at once. For example, one Dr. Gunn, though hardly in the vanguard of his time's medical thinking, was the author of an extremely popular medical guide. At one point in this guide, he calls acute and chronic rheumatism two different diseases ("inflammatory rheumatism" and "chronic rheumatism"); in the second half of the same sentence, however, he calls them different phases of the same disease. Similarly, in one sentence he calls "venereal disease" a single disease, noting that "it took its name from a Greek word, which in our language means FILTHY"; yet he goes on to call syphilis and gonorrhea separate diseases in their own right.[8]

These statements are not so contradictory as they may seem on the surface. Consider that, for Dr. Gunn, the pattern needed to call something a disease rarely involved common origins (such as germs or poisons), most of which were difficult if not impossible to identify anyway, given the technology of the time; instead, a disease pattern generally involved symptoms or groups of symptoms. Consequently, some of Dr. Gunn's decisions to call certain phenomena diseases seem ludicrous today. For example, one of the diseases listed in *Gunn's Domestic Medicine* is called "drinking cold water when over-heated." Gunn documents five persons in New York who expired from "this fatal disease" in less than ten minutes "from drinking cold water":

> In truth, the deaths became so frequent at the different watering places throughout the town, that placcards [sic] or printed bills were ordered by the CITY COUNCIL to be

stuck up on the different pumps, to caution all persons against drinking cold water when over-heated, or in too large quantities.[9]

Today's readers might ask what caused Gunn to interpret this phenomenon as one unique disease. Most of us would likely come up with a very different explanation. Maybe each of the five persons Gunn mentioned had what we today would consider a different disease: one had a heart condition and had been running; one was merely "out of shape" and overstrained the heart; one was about to die of cancer anyway; and so on. True, they all had one thing in common—a drink of cold water before the final moment—but this one act hardly gave them the same "disease." Or maybe each water pump infected each victim in a different way—one with a poison, another with typhoid germs, and so forth. Instead of focusing on these other possibilities, however, Gunn chose an understandable explanation, given contemporary knowledge of germs and heart disease: the water and its coldness. Dr. Gunn and his contemporaries may also have been inspired by a similar phenomenon seen in the then-ubiquitous horse, for stable owners today report that horses will often "drop dead" if they drink cold water when overheated.

▲ THE DREAM OF NOSOLOGY

As the disease "drinking cold water when over-heated" suggests, criteria used to distinguish one disease from the next have changed over time. Entities once distinguished by obvious and visible manifestations—such as asthma—or by clusters of obvious manifestations—such as gout or diabetes mellitus—have been reclassified according to completely different features, most not observable to an old-fashioned doctor sitting at the patient's bedside. Doctors in the early nineteenth century began to distinguish diseases by looking at the lesions produced inside a patient's body instead of considering his coughs, colors, and cries. Or they looked at a disease's microbiology or biochemistry, rather than the patient's odor, as the distinctive mark of a disease.[10]

These changes can be traced back to the eighteenth century, a time when many doctors were trying to find a way to sort out the many new diseases then being discovered. The desire to classify diseases—a task known as nosology—grew out of the more general desire to classify all natural phenomena. Sixteenth-century scientists had organized plants and animals into genera and species, classifying rocks and trees and herbs, birds and fish and beasts. Of course, even ancient Greek scientists had classified data, but the rate of discovery after the Renaissance made the need for classification much more pressing: the human mind cannot contend with masses of unorganized facts and somehow needs to systematize them. It was obviously inefficient to look at each new patient as a wholly new phenomenon, dealing with each illness from scratch and drawing nothing from accumulated experience. Classification of diseases would allow doctors to relate the experience of one patient to the experiences of other patients; it would be possible to know exactly what would work and would not work without having to rely on trial and error.

Consequently, the English physician Thomas Sydenham (1624–1689) proposed a classification scheme based on a complete picture of each disease. Sydenham believed that a disease was not just a generalized imbalance or weakness, but, rather, a definite entity which followed very specific principles.[11] In other words, all people with the same disease shared certain symptoms and certain internal damage, just as all plants of the same species shared the same general leaf and stem structure.

One of the ways Sydenham showed the distinctness of each disease was to discuss the efficacy of quinine. Explorers had recently brought *quinaquina* bark back from Peru, and Sydenham found that patients treated with this substance recovered from ague (malarial fever) without the usual treatments. Sydenham argued that the quinine had a very specific effect on this particular disease, and he urged future physicians to aim at finding similar specific remedies for other diseases.[12] He also advocated defining specific diseases by linking observable symptoms with inner damage to organs and tissues.

Given the state of medical knowledge during the seventeenth and eighteenth centuries, however, that goal was more easily stated than achieved. Not that people didn't try. In 1734, François Boissier de Sauvages de la Croix (1706–1767), the most famous medical nosologist, published a preliminary study, which he completed with a monumental work in 1763.[13] One of his correspondents, the Swedish botanist and physician Carl von Linné (Linnaeus), known as the father of botanical classification, simultaneously attempted to classify human diseases in his *Genera Morburum* (1763).[14] But neither Linnaeus nor any of his contemporaries could come up with a perfect system. One of the major problems had to do with deciding exactly which criterion (which "clincher") would be used to distinguish one disease from the other.[15]

Would it be symptoms? Causes? Location? One nosologist even considered using the letter of the alphabet that started a disease's name to separate groups of diseases.

Even among those nosologists who used the same criterion, however, contradictory systems emerged. For example, although both Linnaeus and Boissier de Sauvages used symptoms and signs (usually) to define specific disease, Linnaeus ended up with eleven classes of disease whereas Boissier de Sauvages arrived at ten. And later, when the British physician William Cullen (1710–1790), the author of an eighteenth-century work on nosology and a leading medical thinker of his time, used symptoms to distinguish diseases, he wound up with only four classes. Worse still, whereas Linnaeus defined 325 different diseases in this way, Boissier de Sauvages defined 2,400![16] Many of Boissier de Sauvages' "diseases" were what we today would consider symptoms, but, given the limited understanding of etiology at the time, his confusion is understandable.

Using cause as the criterion worked no better, again because so little was known about disease causation that such schemes often reflected talented imaginations more than empirically grounded deductions. Erasmus Darwin (1731–1802), the grandfather of Charles, for example, devoted one volume of his ambitious work *Zoonomia* to classifying disease by causal factors. For Darwin, all illness stemmed from either an excess or a deficiency of some sort. Unfortunately, Darwin therefore concluded that merely identifying the excess or deficiency was equivalent to identifying the cause. To say that a catarrh is "caused" by excess mucous secretion is not very helpful: the catarrh *is* the excess mucous secretion. In other words, Darwin often used the definition of a disease or symptom in lieu of its cause.[17]

Neither type of eighteenth-century classification system is at all useful today. Because these systems were fundamentally based on what we consider to be symptoms, they are little more than lists and never suggest a particular course of a disease based on a particular set of symptoms. Consequently, for modern physicians these nosologies, besides being contradictory, have little predictive power. It is important to understand, however, that for the doctors drawing them up they *were* useful: any disease that Linnaeus classified as "exanthemata" (fever with spotty skin eruptions), for example, could be expected to have a different course and treatment than a disease classified as "critical fever" (a fever in which the urine shows a red sediment). These classifications mean little to us today, but for Linnaeus they provided a way to distinguish one group of patients from the next.

Similarly, practicing physicians of the eighteenth and early nineteenth centuries used symptoms alone to define a pattern and thereby labeled many conditions as "diseases" in a way that seems strange to us today—including "suppression, or stoppage of urine," "eating snuff," "sore eyes," and, of course, Dr. Gunn's "drinking cold water when overheated." Sometimes they were not even talking about patterns but were simply using the term "disease" in a very primitive sense, to mean dis-ease. More often, though, when physicians spoke of "disease" they meant a full-fledged pattern, albeit a very different pattern than we would generally accept today. These patterns were also less rigid than today's. One disease (i.e., a set of symptoms) could change into another, and the mind could influence this change as much as any physical event; for example, grief or greed—or "moral" inadequacies—could make your stomach ache or your head burn.[18]

Anatomy as Clincher

The belief that every disease represents a distinct entity and follows its own distinct laws continued into the nineteenth century, even if the classification schemes continued to differ. Because medical technology had grown, however, Sydenham's dream of linking external symptoms to internal lesions was becoming more of a reality. Particularly in Paris, researchers were defining an array of new diseases by comparing their clinical experience with postmortem examinations of the same patients. Newer classification schemes therefore could use a presumably more fundamental characteristic of a disease; instead of assuming that all fevers belong in the same category, for example, doctors could link up certain fevers with different diseased organs (the intestine, say, or the windpipe) and thus consider them separate diseases. By looking at *internal anatomical changes* in order to distinguish medical disorders, doctors could now disentangle previously intertwined diseases.[19]

Improved imaging and staining techniques allowed researchers to be even more specific when identifying diseases. As the nineteenth century progressed, researchers in France and, a bit later, in England realized that, for many conditions, it was not the specific location or organ that distinguished a disease, but rather the specific *tissue* affected; for example, an inflammation of the skin was a different disease than an inflammation of the mucous membranes or an inflammation of the muscles and joints.[20] The key was always to link up the internal change with the external symptoms.

Many years later, when researchers could distinguish changes in cells and, eventually, in molecules, they likewise tried defining diseases along these even more specific lines. Sickle-cell anemia, for example, is a disease identified by an aberration in one part of the hemoglobin molecule. However sophisticated, all of these examples illustrate an attempt to define and classify diseases according to an aberration in some specific anatomical locale—whether that locale be an organ, a tissue, a cell, or a molecule.

The Move to Nosography

Toward the end of the eighteenth century, some doctors began to despair of finding a perfect classification for all diseases. More useful, men like Philippe Pinel (1745–1826) argued, would be devising a complete description of each disease—a pursuit known as nosography. While the move away from strict genus and species meant more flexibility, nosography did imply classification in a sense, for merely naming a disease implies some sort of classification.[21] To give a disease a name means that it has been separated out somehow from other diseases, perhaps not classified in a universal scheme but nonetheless classified as a distinct entity.

The search for a universally recognized medical nomenclature also spurred on the separation of one disease from the next. The *Manual of the International Statistical Classification of Diseases, Injuries, and Causes of Death* defines "medical nomenclature" as a list or catalog of approved terms for describing and recording clinical and pathological observations.[22] To derive such terms, physicians have to decide from many observed conditions just what elements are essential to each disease, a decision believed crucial to medical progress by modern physicians. According to the historian Gerald Grob, for example, one resolution introduced at the first meeting of the National Medical Convention (which in 1847 became the American Medical Association) urged the medical profession to agree on a nomenclature of diseases in order to enhance the utility of registration categories. "The absence of a clearly stipulated nomenclature was an insuperable barrier," notes Grob. "Often the same disease went under a variety of names; and accurate comparisons of the prevalences of disease or health of the population in different places and periods were impossible."[23]

As the nineteenth century progressed, new methods gave investigators the ability to correlate symptoms not just with abnormal-looking internal parts, but with abnormally working internal parts. In other words, it was now possible to correlate physiology (the functioning of the body) with what a doctor saw in the clinic. This kind of linkage became easier with tools like the stethoscope, which allowed clinicians to learn something about how well the heart was functioning inside the patient and to compare that with simultaneous symptoms on the outside.

Meanwhile, in Germany, improved microscopic and chemical power also allowed a whole generation of German clinicians to learn something about the malfunctioning of organs and cells. Metabolic and endocrinological conditions like diabetes and thyroid disorders suddenly became understandable as full-fledged diseases: they represented the malfunctioning of various bodily systems which, presumably, could be linked with some organic lesion or disease.[24] German investigators talked about disorders such as "cardiac insufficiency," "ventricular insufficiency," and "intestinal insufficiency"—disorders defined not by a particular symptom or internal lesion, but by a specific malfunction of the heart, stomach, or intestines. Sometimes this view was taken to great extremes; one researcher, for example, even considered such functional disorders as excessive secretion of acid by the stomach ("hyperacidity") as specific diseases.[25]

Just like the nosologists before them, many of these physiological investigators thought that they had finally latched onto the real essence of disease, even if they no longer were overtly trying to construct neat nosologies. If doctors could only "catch" the malfunctioning physiological process, patch up the leaky vessel, soothe the misbeating heart—before the anatomical damage was caused—disease could be stopped at the root.

The mistake these researchers made was assuming that the malfunction represented the true "root" of the disease. They believed that if you just repaired the physiology, the anatomical changes and other symptoms would clear up or would never appear in the first place. In many instances, however, the lesion was more fundamental than the disturbed physiology. For example, mitral valve stenosis (an abnormally narrow valve between the upper and lower left chambers of the heart) may lead to a heart murmur. What needs fixing here is the valve, not the murmur, which itself is only a sign of a more fundamental anatomical problem. Furthermore, the same physiological disturbance could represent several different diseases: a heart murmur can signal any one of dozens of forms of heart disease. Thus, although using dysfunction as a clincher helped doctors better understand certain conditions—especially if no one could identify a deeper cause or a fundamental lesion—disturbed function was no more the clincher that allowed doctors to distinguish every disease than were symptoms or anatomical lesions.[26]

Further technological improvements led investigators to unravel yet another way to separate diseases: heredity. By 1803, researchers had noticed that hemophilia tended to run in families, and by the mid-nineteenth century they had noticed a similar pattern for color blindness, although there was no way to explain how such conditions could arise. Only with the growth of genetic theory in the early twentieth century did researchers begin systematically to investigate diseases that could be distinguished chiefly by some unique pattern inherited in the genes.[27]

From Symptoms to Etiology

None of these methods of distinguishing one disease from the next—symptoms, lesions, dysfunction, or genetics—truly satisfied doctors. Each worked well enough for certain diseases, but none worked for all. Although no one really believed anymore that diseases could be classified like plants and animals, they did want to be able to organize diseases in some coherent fashion by describing them thoroughly. Such organization would mean a better understanding of disease and, ultimately, more logical treatment. There was a sense that by describing diseases, a truly fundamental criterion would emerge to distinguish them.

For many doctors, the obvious criterion was cause or, more precisely, etiology. Physicians had maintained for years that what truly made a disease unique was some distinctive cause; therefore, by preventing or removing this cause they could prevent or remove the disease. The difficulty had always been finding the cause.

In the latter part of the nineteenth century, however, that difficulty was evaporating with respect to certain infectious diseases. Physicians had isolated specific bacteria and associated them with specific diseases, and many claimed that a true cause had been found at last. Finally it was possible to pull apart the many conditions previously lumped together. Typhoid fever was truly unique from other conditions because only typhoid fever was "caused by" the typhoid bacillus. Diphtheria was truly unique because it was "caused by" the diphtheria bacillus. Cholera was truly unique because it was "caused by" the cholera bacillus. Other conditions may have involved identical symptoms or lesions or dysfunctions, but without the unique bacillus—the clincher—the patient did not have any of the foregoing diseases.

At the same time, knowing the etiology of a disease also allowed doctors to lump together conditions they had previously thought of as distinctive. For example, after Robert Koch (1843–1910) had linked the tubercle bacillus to tuberculosis, doctors realized that conditions such as catarrh and scrofula were not separate diseases at all; rather, they were forms of tuberculosis. Similarly, only after the discovery of the spirocheta pallida could investigators conclusively prove that general paralysis and tabes were actually aspects of syphilis. Suddenly it made sense how there could be many different forms or phases of one disease: they all had the same origin.

Despite these achievements, even etiology had its problems as the grand criterion. For one thing, although many infectious diseases were falling into place, a number of diseases could not be classified according to etiology. Thus, noninfectious diseases such as Graves' disease or Bright's disease, which involved abnormal functioning of the thyroid gland and kidney, respectively, appeared to be distinct diseases and yet had no known causes.[28] Furthermore, even for infectious diseases, labeling "cause" soon turned out to be a lot more complicated than just naming a microorganism. In 1884, the German investigator Friedrich Loeffler (1852–1915) isolated the diphtheria bacillus in the throat of a well person. Then, in 1893, investigators at the New York City Health Department detected the diphtheria bacillus in the throats of some perfectly healthy children. They called these children "well carriers" because they carried a disease organism but remained healthy. Investigators meanwhile were finding well and convalescent carriers of other infectious diseases.

Further research also showed that there were different strains of disease-associated bacteria, only some of which might be virulent enough to provoke a specific disease. In other cases, researchers found that unless a person harbored a critical number of the bacteria, no disease would result. This number might vary from person to person. Furthermore, some people seemed to be born resistant to certain diseases or acquired a resistance later in life.[29] It was obviously far too simplistic, therefore, to say that the diphtheria bacterium "caused" diphtheria or that the typhoid bacterium "caused" typhoid fever.

In fact, although harboring a specific infectious organism was a prerequisite for developing a specific disease, it was hardly sufficient. A person's current health and immunological status, based on his genetic construction or life experiences, also played a role in whether or not he would develop a specific disease.[30] Thus, just knowing the etiology of a disease did not necessarily define the disease. Harboring the diphtheria bacillus is not the same as having diphtheria, but it's a necessary part of diphtheria and may induce it in people who are immunologically predisposed. Similarly, overeating is not the same thing as obesity, but it's a necessary part of certain kinds of obesity and may induce it in certain people predisposed by genetics (other forms of obesity may have nothing to do with overeating, however). In other words, just naming a particular predisposition, etiology, symptom, lesion, or dysfunction cannot distinguish each disease from every other disease. There is no one "clincher."

▲ CLASSIFICATION IN ITS PLACE

Without a clincher, then, how do doctors divide one disease from the next? How do they know which of all the varied complaints out there in the world deserve to have a common name? One of the most vivid answers I can recall comes from a biology laboratory experiment that I participated in as a college student. We were studying the taxonomic chart, and by way of explaining classification, the instructor gave us a bag filled with a dozen or so small objects. These objects came in different shapes, sizes, colors, and materials. Each supposedly represented an animal, but that was irrelevant. What we had in front of us were dozens of objects: plastic stars in red, blue, and gold; white metal paperclips, large and small; white plastic squares, large and small; red, blue, and gold rubber bands; red and blue pencils.[31] We were supposed to devise ways to organize all these objects into order, class, genus, and species; that is, along the lines of a standard taxonomic chart. That was all we were told: organize them.

Tables 1, 2, and 3 show some of the schemes my classmates came up with. Obviously, all three schemes successfully place each object in some sort of order, although no single scheme is entirely satisfactory. A perfect scheme would use the same criterion repeatedly to distinguish and lump together the various objects. For example, such a scheme might use function as its single criterion, or perhaps function and other characteristics having some bearing on function. This scheme would be ideal because using it we would know that objects classified near each other have similar functions, while objects classified far from each other have very different functions.

Of course, if we wanted to acquire information about color, this "ideal" functional scheme would be almost useless. For that task, a

Table 1 ▲ ***Mary's Scheme***

Order	Class	Genus	Species
OFFICE SUPPLIES	holders	rubber bands	red rubber bands, gold rubber bands, blue rubber bands
		clips	large paperclips, small paperclips
	writers		blue pencils, red pencils
DECORATIVE OBJECTS	stars		red plastic stars, blue plastic stars, gold plastic stars, white plastic stars
	squares		large white squares, small white squares

scheme based on color alone would be ideal, because it would indicate that objects near each other had similar colors. Such consistent classification schemes are desirable, then, because they are most useful—that is to say, we can derive concrete information from them.

In contrast to such ideal arrangements, my classmates' schemes seem somewhat arbitrary in the features chosen as criteria. In Mary's view (Table 1), plastic is not an important feature for dividing the objects, whereas in Jeff's (Table 2) it is the chief criterion. In Mary's scheme, function is a fairly consistent criterion for dividing, whereas in Jeff's it is color. In Lynn's (Table 3) it is sometimes function, sometimes material, and sometimes appearance that determines placement.

The objects that the class received in the laboratory, however, had been chosen purposely to defy any ideal, wholly consistent classification scheme. I know, because no matter how many hours I spent shuffling and reshuffling objects, I kept running into the same impediments as Mary, Lynn, and Jeff. Most of the class chose fairly obvious divisors—considering color, size, function, material, and shape. We might have considered weight or place of origin or first initial of the object's name as well, but these criteria seemed less logical. Besides,

Table 2 ▲ *Jeff's Scheme*

Order	Class	Genus	Species
PLASTIC	white	squares	small white plastic squares, large white plastic squares
		stars	white plastic stars
		red	red plastic stars
		blue	blue plastic stars
		gold	gold plastic stars
RUBBER		red	red rubber bands
		blue	blue rubber bands
		gold	gold rubber bands
METAL			large paperclips, small paperclips
WOOD			red pencils, blue pencils

even when I tried to be more creative, I still couldn't come up with one method that seemed uniquely useful and informative.

But all that was irrelevant, the instructor told us. The point of the exercise was not to discover one perfect arrangement, but to show that many arrangements were possible and that none was perfect for all purposes.[32] To illustrate this, our instructor asked us to imagine that Mary, Lynn, and Jeff had used their schemes to organize a small shop. Each student divided the shop into sections according to the "order" category: thus, Lynn and Jeff each had four sections (red, white, blue, and gold for Lynn and plastic, rubber, metal, and wood for Jeff), whereas Mary had only two (office supplies and decorative objects). Each section held a counter for each "class" of objects, and each "genus" took up one shelf of the appropriate counter. Each "species" lay in its own box on these shelves.

Next the instructor asked the class to imagine a new clerk working in these shops. A customer comes in, wanting "something to hold

Table 3 ▲ **Lynn's Scheme**

Order	Class	Genus	Species
RED		toys	red stars
		office supplies	red rubber bands, red pencils
WHITE	squares	plastic	large white plastic squares, small white plastic squares
	clips	metal	large white metal paperclips, small white metal paperclips
	stars		white plastic stars
BLUE		toys	blue plastic stars
		office supplies	blue rubber bands, blue pencils
GOLD			gold rubber bands, gold plastic stars

papers together." What questions would the new clerk have to ask in order to satisfy the customer and sell the merchandise? We looked at the three shops and answered. In Lynn's shop, we decided, the dialogue would go something like this:

> **Clerk:** How can I help you, Ma'am?
> **Customer:** I'd like something to hold my papers together, please.
> **Clerk** *[looking at the four sections]:* Would that be red, white, blue, or gold, Ma'am?
> **Customer:** To be quite honest, I couldn't care less. I'd just like something to hold my papers together.
> **Clerk** *[beginning to sweat]:* Well, let's take a look. *[They walk over to the red section, where there is one case and two shelves—toys and office supplies.]* I suppose that would be on the office supplies shelf.
> **Customer:** That sounds reasonable.

> **Clerk** *[looking at the red rubber bands and red pencils on the shelf]:* Well, here we go then. The rubber bands should do the trick.
>
> **Customer:** I suppose. But clips or binders are more what I was thinking of. Do you have any?
>
> **Clerk:** I don't know. Let's check the other sections . . .

And so on. By now, we were tired; and we were sure the customer was, too. There had to be a better way.

Indeed, there was. Look what happened when the same customer went into Mary's shop, a place with an equally inexperienced clerk:

> **Clerk:** Hello. How can I help you today?
>
> **Customer:** I'd like something to hold my papers together, please.
>
> **Clerk** *[looking at the sections]:* Of course. Let's go to the office supplies section. *[They do so and find two cases, one labeled "holders," the other labeled "writers." The clerk walks over to the case of holders and surveys the shelves: rubber bands and paper clips.]* Would you prefer rubber bands or clips?
>
> **Customer:** Clips, please.
>
> **Clerk:** Large or small?
>
> **Customer:** Oh, give me a few of each.

And the sale was made! Lynn blushed and hung her head. It looked like Mary would get an A on the assignment. But then the instructor asked us to consider what would happen if a customer came into Mary's store wanting "something stretchy for fixing the propeller on a toy helicopter." Here's what we came up with:

> **Clerk:** Hello. How can I help you, sir?
>
> **Customer:** I need something stretchy to fix the propeller on my son's toy helicopter. Any ideas?
>
> **Clerk** *[looking at the sections]:* Would those be office supplies or decorative objects?
>
> **Customer** *[shrugging]:* I don't know. My son just told me the propeller doesn't turn anymore.

Clerk: Hmm. I don't know if we have them then. We only carry office supplies and decorative objects.
Customer: All right then. Thank you. I'll try across the street.

Actually, a simple rubber band would have solved this customer's problem, and even though the clerk had rubber bands in stock, he lost the sale. Because the customer was thinking in terms of "toys," the idea that something for fixing toys might be found in the office supplies section never occurred to him or to the clerk.

In the meantime, the disappointed customer goes across the street, this time to Jeff's shop. Here he finds things a lot easier:

Clerk: Hi there. What can I do for you today?
Customer: Something stretchy. I see you have a rubber section.
Clerk [looking around]: Yes, indeed. [They walk into the rubber section, and, seeing rubber bands, the customer's eyes light up.] Any particular color?
Customer: I like red. Do you have any red rubber bands?
Clerk [looking in the red case and seeing only red rubber bands]: Here we go. A whole box.
Customer: Terrific. I'll take a dozen—that should keep the kid happy for months.

By this time the nature of the problem was clear to us, and we didn't have to rehearse similar dialogues for different customers in all of the shops. We could see that some schemes worked well for some purposes but were cumbersome for others. Furthermore, we saw that a scheme could actually ruin a sale by excluding certain terms. Thus, when the customer wanting something stretchy for a toy came into Mary's shop, he assumed the store didn't carry this item because the sections were labeled "office supplies" and "decorative objects." A "rubber" section in another store, however, was all he needed to trigger the idea of rubber bands and make his purchase. From this exercise, then, we learned several things applicable to the classification of diseases as well as objects:

1 Most schemes are imperfect because they use no single criterion for dividing items.

2 Different arrangements can be useful in one context and cumbersome in another.
3 What is considered an order or a class in one scheme may be considered a mere genus in another. Although the items to be classified stay the same from scheme to scheme, the emphasis varies.

If you substitute the word "disease" for "order," and the term "patient experience" for "species" in these schemes, you will begin to understand the meaning of disease in our society. I mean this only metaphorically. No one has seriously attempted to equate diseases with categories on a taxonomic table for centuries. In a very loose sense, however, this metaphor suggests the transience of disease names and explains why there can be no one clincher that explains how we differentiate one disease from the next. In the taxonomic scheme, the only "material" or "real" things are the species—the red plastic stars, the gold rubber bands, and the like. The other terms— "office supplies," "metal," or "red," for example, are abstractions (like Platonic forms) applied to groups of objects. It is now clear that these abstract terms can vary and that by changing the classification scheme, orders (like diseases) come and go.

It's crucial to remember, then, that what we mean by a "disease" varies with time and place; it is merely a *model,* useful in considering certain known phenomena. This model is useful because it gives structure to otherwise random information and tells us that if we see A, it was probably caused by B and will result in C. We talk in terms of diseases only because, by grouping together certain characteristics into patterns—coherent constellations of symptoms, specific causes, and specific outcomes—we can better predict or explain certain events. Clearly it has been useful to think of "diphtheria," "diabetes," and "multiple sclerosis" when studying new treatments, advocating patient care, and finding (and therefore potentially eliminating) causes.

Nothing is inherently distressing in this process; in fact, creating order out of chaos is the basic task of the scientist. In medicine, the danger lies in premature naming with respect to individual patients— which leads to inappropriate treatment and faulty research—and in forgetting that we must revise our disease models as the state of the art changes. As soon as the model stops being useful, as soon as experience contradicts the theory, the model must be rejected.

When should we make that decision to reclassify conditions? When should we decide what criteria are relevant or not? As we have seen, there is no absolute answer; nonetheless, these decisions must be made. What we are left with, then, is convenience or expedience— Is it useful to think of these sets of conditions as one disease or not? Do they have enough in common to justify thinking of them in the same category? Or does such a grouping cause more confusion than it's worth? For every condition, these questions must be answered, and rather subjectively. There is no neat scheme. Nor should there be: a medical science that would constantly adjust to new discoveries requires this very ambiguity. The price we must pay, however, is constant vigilance.

▲

CHAPTER 4

Are There Really Any Diseases?

▲ FALLING THROUGH THE CRACKS

Years ago my Uncle Jerry decided to do something about a strange growth on the bottom of his foot. His doctor identified it as a plantar wart—a common wart that becomes imbedded in the bottom of the foot by pressure—and recommended burning it off with an electrical wire. This was a standard procedure for removing plantar warts and should have done the trick. It didn't, though. The wart returned, and another doctor tried to burn it off. Still, the stubborn plantar wart returned. A third and fourth visit to a doctor included applying acid to the wart as well, all to no avail. For the time being, then, my uncle decided to live with it.

After living with this growth for several more years, however, my uncle found himself in the hospital for minor surgery. His surgeon suggested that while he was doing the surgery, he might as well remove the persistent plantar wart once and for all. Because the surgery this time was done in the hospital, rather than in the doctor's office, the excised wart was sent to the pathology lab to be studied. Lo and behold, the hospital pathologist soon announced that this was not a plantar wart at all, but an ordinary corn that happened to have been pressed into the sole of the foot. Corns are pea-sized areas of thickened skin, which usually appear on the toes. Indeed, because it was so rare to find a corn on the sole of the foot, the surgeon wrote up the case for a prestigious medical journal ("Patient GW, age 33") and described this growth as a new variant of corn.

According to my uncle, lots of people had corns on the soles of their feet, but whenever such growths appeared on the sole they were misclassified as plantar warts simply because no one ever recognized that anything except plantar warts could occur there. Usually doctors could distinguish a wart from a corn or a callus by scraping it and examining the underlying structure, but clearly my uncle's previous doctors had found it difficult to eyeball a little round growth implanted in the sole of his foot. Instead, his doctors had simply assumed what all outward appearances suggested. When the wart didn't "behave" like normal plantar warts by disappearing after excision, they simply assumed that they hadn't got it all out or that my uncle had an especially persistent wart, rather than considering that they might have given it the wrong name in the first place. In truth, the only thing that was going to keep the growth from recurring was a better-fitting pair of shoes.

Although frustrating, my uncle's case pales before that of K., an unfortunate patient described in the 1981 book *Medical Choices, Medical Chances.* When K. was only eighteen months old, his mother brought him to the hospital with an ear infection. The staff soon recognized a vast array of additional problems, not least of which was a mother who apparently forced him to eat by shoving potato chips, jar baby food, and skim milk—virtually his only foods—down his throat and holding his mouth closed until he swallowed. He was emaciated, pale, and withdrawn and also had some sort of immune deficiency that impaired his ability to fight off infections.

The hospital staff's response to K. was a desperate desire to diagnose his disease. They absolutely refused to treat the child's severe malnutrition until they knew specifically what was wrong with him, and so they subjected him to needles in the arm, the neck, and the spine, desperately trying to find a name for the disease. Upset even further by all the poking and probing, K. not surprisingly still refused to eat. One intern, however, bucked the establishment and tried to take the case into his own hands. He decided to end the disturbing diagnostic tests and simply tried to feed the child, observing that until then, the only emotional reaction K. ever got was his mother's anger at his not eating. Not only did the intern hope that positive feedback would encourage the child to eat, but he suspected that better nutrition might also help alleviate K.'s infections.

The intern's "experimental treatment" was working moderately well until he went on vacation. As soon as K. spiked a fever, the hospital staff ran more tests. The result? Still no diagnosis, but when the intern returned he had to start all over again with an angry and recalcitrant child. As he faced the end of his six-week rotation in that ward, he decided to transfer K. to the psychiatric ward, where at least there was some understanding that emotions play a role in therapy. But there, too, as soon as K. developed a fever, the staff, fearful of ignoring a physical problem, returned him to the main, acute-care ward. Another battery of invasive tests, with needles and tubes stuck into all available orifices, revealed nothing decisive, and this time K. became extremely depressed. His malnutrition worsened, and—despite an intravenous line to pump in calories—K. had been so severely weakened by the combined effects of constant infection, starvation, and medical testing that soon afterward he turned blue and died.[1]

As the authors point out, K.'s condition almost certainly represented the cumulative result of a variety of problems, including malnutrition, emotional neglect, and possibly some kind of immunodeficiency. But the desperate desire to name, to squeeze the sick child into a single category instead of accepting that his peculiar pattern of problems fell between the definitional cracks, blinded doctors to the possibility that it might be feasible to treat a patient without categorizing him.

▲ TWO VIEWS OF ILLNESS

This tendency to shove all new observations into a predetermined scheme—and to overlook any condition that falls between the cracks—is one of the basic problems that comes from sticking too closely to any classification scheme. If your condition happens to fall between the cracks of the established system of names, as did the corn on my uncle's foot, your condition may receive the wrong name and, therefore, the wrong treatment—or, like K., you may receive no treatment at all. This phenomenon stems from seeing a disease name as a hard-and-fast category, true for all time; this view of disease can be traced back many centuries.

Throughout history, in fact, doctors have viewed illness in one of two basic ways: 1) as a manifestation of one of many distinct bodily afflictions or 2) as an imbalance in the body's normal functioning. Philosophers of medicine have called the first view "ontological" and the second "physiological."[2] In the physiological view, all illness represents a variation on a theme, and there are no distinct diseases. For ancient Greek physicians, for example, people were healthy if their four bodily "humors" (blood, phlegm, yellow bile, and black bile) were in equilibrium. When the balance between these four fluids was disturbed, disease or illness resulted. This disease was not a distinct "thing" that entered a part of the body but an altered state of the person himself. Disease, whatever its specific nature, could therefore be cured by restoring the natural equilibrium, not by removing the disease (for there was no disease to be removed).[3]

Later physicians modified these views, but still spoke of disease as a state of the body that was in opposition to health. The medical historian Lester King has found, for example, that during the sixteenth and seventeenth centuries many medical thinkers saw disease as a sort of generalized bodily dysfunction. For the Neogalenists (whose thought harkened back to the great ancient Greek physician Galen), disease involved a state of the body "contrary to nature" in which functions could not be performed in a natural fashion. For the eighteenth-century physician Friedrich Hoffmann (1660–1742), who thought that the living body followed the laws of mechanics, disease consisted of "a great change and disturbance in the proportion and order of the motions," accompanied by a "striking disturbance of secretions, excretions, and other functions of the living body." And for Hoffmann's contemporary Hermann Boerhaave (1668–1738), a diseased person was one who could not perform "the several actions proper to the human body with ease, pleasure, and a certain constancy" or who could perform them only "with difficulty, pain, and sudden weariness."[4]

Perhaps the most extreme example of this sort of thinking in Western medicine is the system of the American physician Benjamin Rush (1745–1813), who argued that all the afflictions of humankind were caused by only one disease. This disease was characterized by excess tension in the blood vessels, and different degrees of tension prompted different symptoms. To relieve this excess tension, Rush prescribed bloodletting or purging in order to reduce bodily fluids.[5]

Bizarre as these conclusions might seem to us today, the truth is that for the practicing physician, function and usefulness have always been more important than formal divisions in deciding what is a disease: either the patient's body is working satisfactorily or it's not; and if it's not, something has to be done.[6] In fact, today's doctors still think of some diseases as generalized imbalances that throw off function. Thus, diseases such as Cushing's syndrome (which involves an improper balance of corticosteroids) or hypothyroidism (which involves an improper balance of thyroid hormone) can be treated by righting the balance of hormones in the whole body, not by simply eliminating a poison or reactivating an enzyme. And as the medical writer Lynn Payer documents in her book *Medicine & Culture,* West German and French physicians have a rather strong tendency to emphasize disturbances in the body's internal milieu, or "terrain," rather than any specific external agent, as the base of illness.[7]

Furthermore, traditional Chinese medicine, practiced today by many thousands of physicians, rests on the view that illness represents an imbalance of the body's *qi,* or "vital energy." Patients therefore do not have distinct diseases but rather some specific imbalance that manifests itself in a completely unique set of symptoms.[8] The growing acceptance of acupuncture, acupressure, and herbal medicine even among Western practitioners suggests the efficacy obtainable through this view of illness.

Nevertheless, most Americans today are probably much more familiar with the rival view, whereby a disease is the generalized result when one or another entity "enters" a person and causes a problem: the person is healthy; an outside "disease promoter" arrives to alter the patient's body; and the illness is cured by removing that disease promoter. A disease promoter might be a bacterium, for example, or an environment lacking in some essential nutrient. A disease, in this view, is not an individualized state of imbalance, but a personal attribute— an attribute shared by other persons with the same disease.[9] To cure a disease, then, you get the disease or the promoter of that disease out of the body: you may give vitamin C to "get rid of" scurvy, for example, or administer diphtheria antitoxin to "eliminate" diphtheria.

In recent years, people advocating "holistic" and "biocultural" medicine have criticized this view of illness for disregarding the individual and concentrating instead on the disease, as, in fact, it does. Indeed, as our medical problems shift away from infectious disease and toward chronic illness, we may find it more effective once again to think in terms of an individual's unique circumstances rather than in terms of discrete disease entities; chronic illness is hard to fit into standardized categories, given the variety of life experiences that modify each individual's suffering over time.[10] There can be no denying, however, that against some afflictions (such as infectious diseases), traditional biomedical thinking has been tremendously effective.

To some extent, our thinking about disease and about diseases as distinct entities that descend upon the body arose in the nineteenth century when people conducting medical research became separated from the people caring for patients. Researchers began to look at the organs, tissues, and cells (and, later, the microorganisms) associated with diseases, rather than at an individual sick person, and so they started thinking of diseases more in terms of a specific appearance or a specific germ rather than as generalized bodily dysfunction. Still, we know that even the doctors of ancient Cnidus tried to divide illness into many different diseases, although their ideas about what constituted a unique disease were very different from ours.[11]

▲ ESSENTIALISM: THE FATAL FLAW

The ontological view of illness stems from a philosophical assumption that has haunted thinking about disease for centuries, especially since the nosologists started trying to divide all illness into specific diseases. Most of these early taxonomists assumed that the genera and species that they used to classify diseases were *natural,* somehow built into diseases and existing independently of human terminology.[12] This assumption was akin to assuming that the genera and species used to classify plants and animals are inherent in these life-forms, as if, for example, dogs were—by nature—part of the genus *Canis* and part of the species *familiaris.* These people did not simply invent genera and species to explain what they knew at the time; they discovered supposedly built-in natures by considering ancestry and comparing properties.[13] Once identified, therefore, a genus and species could not be modified. If they were correct, they were correct for all time, since they were inherent—an "essence"—in the plant or animal or disease. Belief in an essence allowed doctors to say that Jenny's sneezing and Johnny's coughing were merely different stages of the same essential disease.

One way to think of essence is to think of a human being—say, Abraham Lincoln. At three months, Lincoln looked, felt, and acted very different from Lincoln at thirty years of age. But whether a child or an adult, young or old, this person remained Abraham Lincoln because some enduring essence—his soul or his genes or something—remained the same whatever his physical appearance. Similarly, it's possible to think of a disease as a process with many stages that look different but with some common essence tying all these stages together.

Even when doctors stopped looking for an inherent genus and species for each disease, their desire to define diseases reflected a belief in some sort of essences. They assumed that there was some natural division that separated one disease from the next—even if they didn't quite know what that division was. For many years, as we have seen, they had to rely on symptoms as their best clue because other clues—such as internal lesions, dysfunction, and cause—were simply too hard to find. Often, too, they assumed "cause" was this more fundamental element, which, once discovered, would lead to a perfect classification scheme.

When the psychiatrist Emil Kraepelin (1856–1926), for example, tried for the first time to distinguish "manic-depressive insanity" as a distinct mental disorder, he assumed that illness could be divided into distinct entities, each with a fundamental essence. Such an assumption resembled that of earlier nosologists who had tried to classify bodily disorders: knowledge might be sparse and boundaries shifting, but each disorder represented a distinct entity with a distinct natural history. Many psychiatrists early in the twentieth century hoped that, by categorizing diseases according to symptoms and analyzing them statistically, they eventually would discover a common cause.[14]

Previously, psychiatrists had spoken of different diseases of the mind, including periodic and circular insanity, simple mania, melancholia, and various colorings of mood. Kraepelin, however, regarded them all as part of a single process. "What has brought me to this position," he wrote, "is first the experience that notwithstanding manifold external differences, certain *common fundamental features* yet recur in all the morbid states mentioned."[15] Each patient may experience different symptoms, and a given symptom may change or never appear, but there remains a definite narrow group of disorders, each of varied character, which in association "impress a uniform stamp on all the multiform clinical states." These, he argued, pass over into each other without recognizable borders and may replace each other; therefore, they all constitute the same disorder known as manic-depressive insanity.[16]

Even today's medical textbooks, which are far too sophisticated to use the taxonomic terms "class," "order," "genus," and "species," still assume that each disease has a defining essence. Thus, a glance at the table of contents in a typical medical textbook reveals chapter titles such as "Diseases of the Kidney" and "Diseases Caused by Anaerobic Bacteria." Merely by putting a disease in a given chapter, the authors have classified it.[17] Why group diabetes mellitis as a metabolic disease, for example, and not as a pancreatic disease? Why group malaria as a protozoan disease and not as a blood disease? Each disease in and of itself shares properties with each category, but to put it in a given chapter reflects a decision that one property is more fundamental to the disease's essence than another. The result is an implicit classification system.

As philosophers since the ancient Greeks have pointed out, the trouble with this or any sort of classification system is that it involves abstractions. People may come up with these systems by evaluating concrete objects, but no one object is exactly equivalent to the genus or species assigned to it. In a zoological scheme, for example, Rin Tin Tin is not synonymous with "dog." He is *a* dog, according to criteria drawn from all observed animals that someone chose to call "dogs," but he is not the species "dog." Think of it this way: you can put your hand on *a* dog, but you can never put your hand on "dog." The names we assign to species don't actually exist in the physical world.

Disease classifications are even further removed from concrete objects than animal or plant classifications. At least an individual oak tree being classified is itself a palpable "thing": you can reach out your hand and feel it, you can eyeball it and describe the texture of its bark, you can hold a leaf in one hand and compare it to the leaf of another oak tree. But any individual case of disease is just as intangible as the abstract disease itself. You can touch John who has a cold; you can hear the sneeze, measure the fever, and examine the mucus—but you can't touch the cold. Even the individual cold is a mental construct, and just assigning it a name does not make it a real object with an underlying essence.

Although this idea may seem obvious, we rarely apply it in everyday life. It is all too easy to forget that diseases are merely useful models, not actual objects. This process of acting as though an abstract concept is a concrete thing is known as "reification," and reification can lead to all sorts of misperceptions.[18] Above all, if we reify diseases— that is, if we think of diseases as objects—we start regarding them as unchangeable and eternal, true for all peoples and all times, and we try to fit people and their illnesses into rigid disease categories, chastising those who don't fit. Probably the greatest victims of our tendency to reify diseases are people suffering from the nameless diseases, which often bridge or fall between contemporary disease categories.[19]

Such behavior is antithetical to the constant vigilance required for good medical and scientific thinking. Instead of fitting the patients to the model, we should be fitting the model to the specific patients. Good scientists, after all, are not supposed to change their data to fit their hypothesis, but must change their hypothesis when the data overwhelmingly suggest its inadequacy.

When pressed, of course, few people would bother to defend a claim that "colds" are material things that burrow into people, provoke sneezes, and then go on their merry way. When we think about it at all, we realize that we say "John has a cold, and Jenny has a cold, too," merely because "cold" is a convenient term. John's condition has enough in common with Jenny's to make it useful for us to think of them as examples of a common abstraction. Yet, language itself lulls us into acting as though diseases were real and unchanging objects. For example, we talk about "catching" a cold, "having" a cold, or "getting rid" of a cold; we even "give" our colds to other people.[20] This sort of language helps us to think of diseases as concrete objects and, in turn, as unchangeable and eternal, true for all peoples and all times. Just because a patient's pain cannot be fit into any known disease model, however, doesn't mean that the patient is lying or crazy or that the doctor is stupid: it merely means that our current models of disease are inadequate to explain this particular patient and his complaints.

The much-maligned nineteenth-century French investigator François-Joseph-Victor Broussais (1772–1838) was quick to point out this faulty assumption, borrowed from the classification of plants and animals and applied inappropriately to diseases. Today's practitioners are barely aware of such philosophical issues, but for many nineteenth-century investigators the fundamental question was: "What is a disease?" Broussais held the physiological view of illness: all illness represents a variation on a theme. He objected to the trend he saw in some of his colleagues of describing an array of distinct diseases, each a separate entity following predetermined laws; because no two patients were identical, he argued, no two had the same disease. Instead, various physiological problems could occur to produce, for example, an inflamed lung or a lesioned intestine, and the unique combination of these irritations in a unique person constituted the condition of illness.[21]

Regarding diseases as special beings like plants or animals represented a flawed system of thought that Broussais called "ontology." Ontological thinking in this sense meant that doctors were assuming that diseases existed as real, unchanging, and therefore completely predictable objects. Broussias objected to ontological thinking and noted that the groups of symptoms called "diseases" by his colleagues "are metaphysical abstractions which by no means represent a constant unchangeable morbid condition, and which we cannot be certain of finding in nature."[22]

Many German investigators also shunned the nosography and

nosology of the Parisian School while applauding Broussais and another French physician, François Magendie (1783–1855), who had called pathology "the physiology of the sick man." These investigators—including Theodor Schwann, Jacob Henle, Rudolf Virchow, Hermann Helmholtz, and Emil DuBois-Reymond—tried to consider the patient as a whole and fought against turning diseases into objects.

German investigators attacked "ontology" by pointing out that names of diseases such as dysentery, cholera, and scrofula were not real entities but simply "practical makeshift" ideas borrowed from lay language. In fact, it was impossible to decide where one disease ended and another began; what mattered was the impaired physiology of the individual patient. As a young man, the eminent investigator Rudolf Virchow (1821–1902) wrote endless tracts on this issue to prove that "the subjects of therapy are not diseases but conditions; [and] we are everywhere only concerned with changes in the conditions of life. Disease is nothing but life under altered conditions."[23]

Such views also appeared among American practitioners of the early nineteenth century, perhaps a natural consequence of disease patterns defined primarily by symptoms. In fact, for many practitioners of the day, the cause of the disease didn't matter, nor did the name of the ailment, because (at least in theory) treatment aimed at symptoms of the individual patient rather than at the disease: if you seemed too weak, perhaps the doctor strengthened you with a tonic; if you were "overexcited" (e.g., feverish), perhaps he soothed you by leeching out some of your blood.[24] Ideally, of course, a physician would get to the root of your condition and eliminate it, but if that proved impossible, soothing the symptoms was perfectly acceptable and, for all intents and purposes, eliminated the "disease."

Furthermore, symptomatic patterns were part of a continuum rather than mutually exclusive entities; therefore, one disease could blur into the next. What had been called separate diseases were really just different forms of a single disease, and thus one condition could transform into another. The highly influential Benjamin Rush contended that, in a matter of weeks or months, "pulmonary consumption is sometimes transformed into head-ach [sic], rheumatism, diarrhoea, and mania. . . . The bilious fever often appears in the same person in the form of colic, dysentery, inflammation of the liver, lungs, and brain, in the course of five or six days."[25]

Thus, the actual name of the disease didn't matter so much as the specific problems of the diseased person. A doctor looked at the patient, saw what was wrong with her (i.e., her signs and symptoms), and tried to remedy those problems—by bleeding, purging, or whatever would "right" the system. This required using what the medical historian John Harley Warner calls the "principle of specificity"; it required looking at the patient as a whole—her body, her environment, and her mind—and determining what would restore equilibrium.[26] Consequently, the name of a disease was often irrelevant: so long as the doctor asked the patient when her problems began, what the symptoms were, what her general health was, and the like—looking for the root of the discomfort but not necessarily finding it—he could provide adequate care. For Dr. Rush, the nosological arrangements of diseases "gratify indolence in a physician, by fixing his attention upon the name of a disease, and thereby leading him to neglect the varying state of the system."[27] This mistrust of names trickled down over the next few decades to ordinary practitioners such as Dr. Gunn, who wrote in 1830 that a man "of good common sense and judgment, who enquires about the habits of the patient will, in nine cases of ten, succeed, when mere theorists who prescribe for the *names* of diseases, without understanding them, will absolutely fail."[28]

However much viewing illness as a generalized imbalance may have reflected reality, that perspective ultimately proved to be impractical. All such talk about the individual patient may make this school of physicians seem like great individualists and humanitarians; but, the truth is, it also could make them great barbarians. The logical clinical consequence of this physiological view of illness was nonspecific, palliative therapy, which sometimes amounted to nothing more than letting nature take its course—simply relieving pain or reducing fevers—but which could also involve extreme intervention.[29] Broussais is often best remembered, in fact, for his overzealous bleeding. Since for Broussais all illness resulted from overstimulation, mainly of the stomach, all illness had to be treated by reducing stimulation; that is, by relieving some of the blood pressure. Whereas other doctors might have said that patients had cancer, tuberculosis, syphilis, measles, malaria, or hepatitis, Broussais would say the problem was "gastroenteritis" and that the solution was leeches on the stomach![30]

As it turned out, viable therapies ultimately ended this trend against essentialism, despite its unquestionably valid elements.[31] With the nineteenth century coming to a close, investigators in both France and Germany had showed the world that, whether or not there really were specific diseases, it was useful to think that there were. In particular, these investigators were identifying specific microorganisms as "causes" of specific diseases and, most important, were producing specific antitoxins to cure them. Perhaps diphtheria was not really a separate entity, but there could be no question that when doctors assumed it was and administered the diphtheria antitoxin to the right patients, those patients got well. For many people, there was just no point in arguing over the philosophy of specific diseases any longer. Specific diseases could be cured!

▲ DISEASES AS PRACTICAL TOOLS

The danger, then, lies not in thinking of diseases as specific entities—such thinking, as twentieth-century Western medicine has shown time and time again, can be extremely effective. Even if diseases don't correspond to absolute reality, they are extremely convenient fictions. As the medical philosopher Knud Faber wrote many years ago: "We must . . . once more emphasize that all concepts of disease, like all other concepts denoting species, are human abstractions, not objective entities." Still, he continued, "to the physician who is to live and act in the world, it is necessary to have definite categories of disease to serve as guides and tools."[32]

For many practitioners, therefore, it doesn't really matter whether objectively there is or isn't a disease—the only thing that matters is whether it's useful to think of the patient as having one. Louis Goldman, an obstetrician-gynecologist in Surrey, England, admits that he doesn't know whether PMS is something real or just an excuse for certain neuroses. But the real point, he says, is that in some cases it is useful when treating patients to believe that PMS exists as a bona fide disease:

> If a woman in her middle 30s tells me that, in the last year or two, she has become very "weepy" or moody before her periods, that these episodes are provoked by incidents that would normally not upset her at all, that the onset of the menses generally relieves her symptoms, and that her husband and children can pinpoint the time of the month by her moods, I am disposed to believe that, for her, PMS offers a reasonable diagnosis.

He adds that if "further history-taking and examination fail to elicit a better explanation, treating her on the tentative diagnosis of PMS strikes me as justified."[33]

No, the danger does not lie in acting as though diseases were separate entities but, rather, in assuming the absolute truth of this merely rhetorical system. Unfortunately, it has become almost impossible not to do so. Investigators over the past hundred years have broken down many infectious diseases into relatively neat categories, associating them with unique germs and therefore unique means of prevention and treatment. Once an etiology is established, in particular, it is easy to assume an essence behind each symptom, some sort of soul or spirit underlying what is seen on the surface. In fact, as late-nineteenth-century investigators pegged down etiologies and specific therapies, it was only natural to see a disease as less shifting, as less of a mere abstraction that describes moment-to-moment symptoms. Such discoveries reinforced the idea that diseases were concrete, mutually exclusive entities. It was better to regard typhoid fever as one disease and treat it with chloramphenicol, for example, than to try bleeding the patient as Rush or Broussais might have done. After all, if psychiatrists were willing to think of Kraepelin's shifting, variable disorder "manic-depressive insanity" as a single, natural entity, ultimately united by a single but as yet unknown cause, how much easier it was for Kraepelin's contemporaries to think of diphtheria, a disease largely defined by etiology, as a natural entity!

This view of disease has become ingrained in modern medicine. Dr. Edmund D. Pellegrino, for example, believes that it represents just one more step in a progression toward curing specific diseases rather than restoring wellness per se. He outlines the emergence of specific therapeutics—the fruit of Sydenham's plea for nosology—starting with lime juice for scurvy in 1753 and going through digitalis (1785) for heart failure, morphine (1806) for pain, transfusion (1818) for blood loss, colchicine (1819) for gout, quinine (1820) for malaria, and clover extract (1926) for pernicious anemia. Physicians once defined diseases in terms of observable symptoms and then narrowed their definitions by using organs, tissues, cells, and, finally, genes, notes Pellegrino, adding that this "progress" will continue, with disease definitions growing more and more specific until we can aim therapy at the molecular level. By asserting that the heart of a problem lies in its smallest feature, Pellegrino is following the reductionist direction of most Western medicine—and, indeed, any examination of medical history will show that the defining characteristics of disease have indeed gone from diseased body to diseased organ to diseased tissue to diseased cell to diseased molecule. Furthermore, researchers have acquired phenomenal powers by looking at immunology or genes as the basis for disease.[34]

The fatal flaw of Pellegrino's argument, however, is its assumption that all diseases are ultimately immutable entities and that medical history is simply the tale of their "discovery." Instead, as we have seen, the early advocates of a standard nomenclature recognized that diseases represent an imposition of order on chaos, a way to group together phenomena so as to maximize efficacy of treatment. The notion that medicine will continue to break down each illness into increasingly specific definitions neglects the fact that because there is no true essence of a disease, the most specific definition of a disease is the individual. There is no real core sitting there waiting to be discovered; although we must assume an essence in order to derive a name for a disease, actually to dig beyond our practical assumptions will only cause the ground to crumble beneath us. In fact, by continuing to subdivide each illness ad infinitum, we risk losing the great advantage of defining disease: the ability to group together patients with different backgrounds. We would land right back where medicine first began— surrounded by a bunch of bewildered doctors trying to make something out of a bunch of sick people with individual makeups and environments.

Specifically, if doctors regarded every patient's condition as entirely unique, determined by an individual set of germs, experiences, and genes, then they would have to approach every new patient as a tabula rasa. It would be impossible to rely on experience when deciding how to treat any particular patient. We would have to acknowledge that every case of sickness really does represent a completely unique pattern—each person's sickness involves a unique germ (your flu virus is not my flu virus), a unique etiology (you spent your childhood in Manhattan and I spent mine in Chicago), unique symptoms (your coughs are drier than my coughs)—and, of course, each *person* is unique to begin with.

For many illnesses, however, most of these specificities are essentially irrelevant. For all intents and purposes doctors can regard the germ, the etiology, and the symptoms as identical in all patients; that is to say, they can regard everyone who has the disease as sharing the same pattern and can therefore treat everyone successfully with the same means.

As time goes on, what changes is not the specificity of our classifications, but how we determine this specificity—what we consider to be a reasonable way to separate one disease from the next. In some cases, particularly for noninfectious diseases and other conditions defined simply as patterns of symptoms or signs, a more reasonable way might actually involve getting *less* specific. And, yes, such conditions still exist: hypertension is characterized not by its origin, but simply by high blood pressure; seasonal affective disorder is characterized not by its cause, but by the timing of its symptoms; and epilepsy is characterized not by its roots but by a certain frequency of seizures (although it can be ruled out if a cause is found that implicates some other disease). For these and many other kinds of disease patterns, it may be too simplistic to think in terms of one cause and one cure; in fact, we may not yet understand enough about these diseases to treat them as monolithic, uniform entities.

What is really happening in medicine, then, is not a progression toward increasingly specific definitions, but, rather, a regrouping of the definitions. If our definitions were truly getting more specific, there would be many more diseases today than ever before. Instead, as we have seen again and again, there are just *different* diseases, classified or distinguished differently as knowledge and technology change.[35] There isn't a finite number of diseases; rather, throughout history and across cultures, symptoms are continually reshuffled for the sake of expedience.

Similarly, what one generation regards as a disease may at some point fit better if it is classified as a symptom of some other disease. Other conditions might be better viewed as generalized imbalances rather than being painfully squeezed into the contemporary scheme of distinct diseases.

▲ A 50 PERCENT CHANCE OF A HEART ATTACK

Thinking about a disease as an unchanging entity leads to all sorts of problems. "A predominantly disease-oriented medical person tends toward cookbook medicine," observes the medical historian Robert Hudson. "The disease is something apart from the patient, an invader of sorts. As soon as this physician can assign a diagnostic term to his patient, the next actions are more or less automatic."[36] Such thinking convinces us that having a disease guarantees a predetermined series of events, and the result can be unnecessary terror. Besides the obvious psychological impact that comes from hearing that we have a disease such as AIDS or cancer, these assumptions can also affect the way other people treat us. Many people equate the word "cancer" with "incurable," for example, and therefore deny health insurance or employment to applicants who ever had any form of this condition, even if there has been no sign of trouble for thirty years.

Many babies who develop a form of cancer known as neuroblastoma recover completely and live perfectly normal adult lives. And yet, according to Dr. Steven Friend, a cancer researcher at the Massachusetts Institute of Technology and Massachusetts General Hospital, as healthy adults these people often can't get health or life insurance—unless they lie and deny ever having had cancer.

Moreover, even if you've never actually "had" an active form of a disease but are diagnosed through some kind of genetic or antibody screening test as "presymptomatic," you may be excluded from benefits or employment. Consider people at risk for Huntington's disease, an as yet untreatable degenerative disease characterized by involuntary jerky movements and mental deterioration. If one of your parents had this disease, you have a 50 percent chance of developing it at some point in your life, with symptoms usually beginning between ages thirty and fifty. It is now possible, however, for people at risk to take a test to show whether or not they have a genetic marker predictive of the disease. Although researchers currently believe that almost everyone with a positive test will eventually develop the disease, potential victims may develop it any time between ages seven and eighty-two, noted Nancy Wexler (a clinical psychologist and the codiscoverer of the DNA test used to detect individuals susceptible to Huntington's disease), speaking at a genetics meeting at the Harvard Medical School. No matter, though. If you're a perfectly healthy twenty-two-year-old woman and your test comes out positive for the marker, you will almost certainly find yourself denied life insurance and a job, even though you could well live symptom-free for the next thirty or more years.

At the same genetics meeting, Paul Billings, a physician at the Harvard Medical School, related the story of a man who had been diagnosed as presymptomatic for the genetic disease hemochromatosis, a condition that involves impaired iron storage and that sometimes results in liver cancer. Although this man said he'd never been hospitalized, often ran ten-kilometer races, and had several doctors write letters to insurance companies documenting his good health, nobody would insure him. In short, he felt so badly discriminated against that he said he'd "rather have AIDS."

To avoid such situations, employers and insurance companies— and scared patients for that matter—must realize that disease categories are meant to serve as useful tools. Remembering this simple fact would liberate us all from the psychological and economic bondage that comes when a name is assigned to our complaint. Often without realizing it, practitioners sense this liberation when they give you a prognosis for a specific disease. When my older daughter was nearly fourteen months old, for example, she suddenly developed bacterial meningitis. I was immediately terrified, remembering that both a friend's grandson and a high school classmate had died of that very same disease. I felt great relief, however, when the resident in the emergency room told me that "the chances of this disease being fatal are very small. And the chances of her returning to normal without any severe aftereffects are very good, too. There is a slightly greater chance that she may develop some hearing loss, but with the treatment we're giving her, her chances are still good." The doctor was speaking in terms of probability, not certainty, and although I was still concerned, I remembered immediately that it was wrong to equate the name of a disease with a fixed outcome. Of course, it was hard for me, as it is for most people, to understand fully a "probability"—we think only of our own outcome, which will definitely occur, whatever the odds—but I still felt better knowing that my baby had a chance to live, rather than "knowing" that she would certainly die.

My daughter's experience was typical. No doctor ever absolutely guarantees what will happen to you, because no individual fits perfectly into any category. The only real "conditions" are the patients themselves, not the disease category they have been lumped into. Of course, some of the uncertainty in prediction stems from inadequate treatment (my daughter would have had an extremely high chance of dying if she hadn't been treated properly) or from individualized responses to treatment; even without any treatment at all, every patient has a unique experience, and that uniqueness is reflected in our limited ability to predict another person's future. Everyone has a story of someone with a fatal disease given three weeks to live who then went on to live another ten years. Such events occur because although most (or even all) previously observed people with that disease may have died within a short time, this death-defying person had some hitherto-unnoticed "something" which set him apart. Maybe he didn't really have the fatal disease. Or maybe he did, but it now turns out that the disease needs to be redefined to include the possibility of living ten more years.[37]

Rather than leaving us with a nihilistic relativism, then, viewing diseases as shifting entities and thinking of disease categories as imperfect constructions actually provides great hope. If a sixty-year-old man is diagnosed as having "metastatic prostate cancer, stage IV" and then proceeds to live another thirty years, debility-free no less, it doesn't necessarily mean that the doctor made the wrong diagnosis or that the man is lying about feeling well—it merely means that our current model of prostate cancer doesn't take into account this particular phenomenon.

Even while using rigid schemes to practice medicine, then, doctors must be aware of the imperfect and ephemeral nature of such schemes. They must, for example, recognize that there is no such thing as an actual "cold"; rather, each person has a cold in a slightly different way—he just has enough of the mutually agreed-upon common signs to make the designation "cold" a useful one. The term "cold" means something in the scientist's mind, but there is no real thing that we can pin down and call a "cold." The "truth," in terms of material reality, is that *there are no diseases.*

The term "material reality" is important, however. Many people maintain that abstractions are just as "real" as material objects.[38] But even these people would agree that there is a difference between what we can hold, touch, and feel and what we only can think. A disease falls into the latter category: it is an abstraction, a general *term* describing many diverse events (the patients). Thus, even depressing odds can be viewed as signs of hope, since no matter how bad the predicted chances, no disease category is so perfect that absolutely everyone with that disease will have an identical experience. And so, just because 50 percent of patients with coronary artery disease end up having a heart attack, that does not mean you will. While odds mean quite a bit to doctors and help to ensure reasonable care, they remain odds—nothing but reasonably good guesses. In the end, everyone is a unique case. This is no great, startling revelation. It is implied in a well-known medical aphorism: "There are no diseases, only sick people."

CHAPTER 5

▲

Mistaking Symptoms for Diseases

▲ WHEN A NAME IS NOT A NAME

As we have noted, patients get a tremendous amount of psychological satisfaction when they receive an answer to the question "What's wrong with me, Doc?" Often, they also get a tremendous amount of social satisfaction: because a disease name generally connotes some associated physical or biochemical defect, it keeps others from blaming the victim. Thus, many people are anxious to attribute defects in themselves or their loved ones to some specific disease (and its underlying physical defect) rather than acknowledge craziness, evil, chance, or stupidity.

Comforting as it is to have a name, however, a misplaced label can devastate someone who is already suffering from disease symptoms. In fact, the temptation to find a name is a little like selling your soul to the devil: immediate fulfillment is so great that you can easily ignore the unpleasant consequences. Often patients are so anxious to know what is wrong with them that doctors will offer them an exotic synonym that describes the complaint. The patient will then immediately misinterpret this term to be the name of a disease, when it is merely a shorthand description of the symptom. Although the term may represent states related to diseases, in and of itself it is nothing more than a translation of an everyday word into medical language. For example, a doctor may tell a man who is losing his hair that he has "alopecia" (baldness) or tell a teenager with pain in his ear that he has "ostalgia" (an earache). Although patients may go home satisfied that the doctor has done his job, they also go home mistakenly believing that they have a disease and that the doctor knows some of its characteristics besides its name.

The implications of such behavior hit home several years ago when my elderly grandmother called me up, terrified. For many years she had had trouble with her eyes—chiefly cataracts (opacity of the normally transparent eye lens), which in turn had produced a form of glaucoma (increased pressure within the eye that may impair vision). Because these conditions were destroying her eyesight, her ophthalmologist several years earlier had surgically removed her natural lenses (to see she used special eyeglasses). Even so, she still complained about "pressure" in her eyes and blurry or double vision.

Now, it seemed, she had yet another disease. As she cried and stuttered into the phone, she told me she had just been to the doctor, complaining as she so often did of her eye troubles.

"What happened, Grandma?" I asked.

It was hard to get a coherent reply. "He said there was no cure," she said.

"No cure? For what?"

"On top of everything else, I now have an incurable condition. He said I'm not a candidate for contact lenses or a lens implant, so I'll have double vision or blurry vision—one or the other—the rest of my life."

"Is there really nothing he can do?"

"That's what he says. Listen, Terra, I know you have access to all sorts of medical information. Do you think you could find out if there are any doctors who can cure this thing? Maybe there's someone out there my doctor doesn't know about."

"Well, sure," I said. "What's the name of the disease?"

"Aphakia," she said, spelling it out for me. "*A* as in apple, *p* as in Peter, *h* as in horse . . ."

"Yes, Grandma, I have it. Aphakia." Funny, in all my years of medical writing I hadn't ever encountered that disease. "Listen, I'll do a search on the computer and see what I can come up with."

My grandmother hesitated. "Well, all right. But how long will it take? Is there anything I can do in the meantime? Should I call the American Medical Association?"

"No. Wait until I look into this."

And so, for several days, she waited by the phone as I pressed buttons on my computer to search the voluminous medical literature for cures of this unfamiliar disease, "aphakia." It turned out that there were more than three thousand scientific publications on this subject; but, after narrowing my search to recent studies about "postcataract aphakia" and "aphakia in the elderly," I finally came up with seventeen likely papers.

Before I called my grandmother, however, so that she could ask her doctor about these papers, I did something I should have done to begin with—I looked up "aphakia" in my medical dictionary. And suddenly I understood why I had never heard of this disease before. Aphakia wasn't a disease at all, but merely a term that meant "absence of a lens." That was something my grandmother could have told you about herself.

From that, I pieced together the scenario in the doctor's office. My grandmother came in periodically to complain about her blurred and double vision, and the doctor kept telling her that there was nothing he could do about it. She had had these problems since her surgery; nothing had changed. But because she did not have a name attached to her condition, she was dissatisfied. She kept pushing the doctor, asking "what" she had, so that she could understand why it couldn't be cured. Perhaps she also said she wanted to ask the medical people in her family about her condition. At last the doctor reached a breaking point, and he told her she had "aphakia" (perhaps among several other "conditions"). She shuddered: she already knew that she "had" cataracts and glaucoma (despite the operation), but this was something new.

"Write that down on a piece of paper for me," she demanded of the doctor. Shaking, she went home, devastated to have yet another disease but also planning to barrage the medical world with requests to cure a disease that didn't even exist—all that time (for me) and agony (for my grandmother) over a phantom.

▲ ANEMIA, HYPOGLYCEMIA, AND OTHER TRICKSTERS

Confusing a synonym for your symptom with a disease is only the most blatant way to confuse symptoms with diseases. At other times, people equate a symptom with something they falsely believe is a disease. For example, a lot of people who feel a little tired now and then decide that their problem is "anemia." They believe that anemia is a disease, and so to cure it they follow a regime prescribed in a popular magazine.

Confusing fatigue with the disease "anemia" amounts to a two-fold error. First of all, even real anemia is not a disease at all; it is a *sign* of any of hundreds of diseases, including tuberculosis, arthritis, kidney failure, sickle-cell anemia, and acute leukemia. Second, although anemia has a very straightforward definition, people with a vast array of symptoms that have nothing to do with this definition keep claiming to have anemia. According to David Steinberg, a specialist in blood diseases, anemia is quite simply a lower than normal amount of hemoglobin—the molecule that transports oxygen—in the red blood cells. People don't "have anemia," then; they have some other disease that produces a specific state of the blood known as anemia.[1]

But many people, regardless of their hemoglobin level, say that they "have anemia." They use "anemia" as if it were the disease that accounted for certain symptoms—especially for feeling lethargic.[2] The reason for this sleight of hand, Dr. Steinberg suspects, is that the name "anemia," which sounds like a disease, is an easy rationalization of fatigue and lack of ambition: "Many people who feel tired and run down find it difficult to accept that their fatigue might be due, for example, to depression and not a physical disease."[3] Somehow, everything that people do, say, or feel becomes justified only if they can attribute their symptoms to an outside force or an identifiable biochemical process. That's where believing you have a disease comes in handy.

The blame for these kinds of mix-ups should not fall entirely in the patient's lap. Doctors are equally tempted into dispensing labels that sound like specific disease names because they know that's what their patients expect; and if you don't do what your patients want, you often end up losing your patients. When Doris went to see her doctor about the dizzy spells she had been having, for instance, the doctor listened to her tell about the three other doctors she had seen. Doris complained about how these doctors "knew less than I did. They couldn't find anything wrong, and so they just sent me home. One guy even told me I was imagining all this and if I just found some meaningful work, I would stop feeling sorry for myself."

Doris's doctor wanted to be sympathetic to his patient, and he said that it sounded like she might have "hypoglycemia." Doris nodded: several of her friends had been talking about hypoglycemia, and that was what she had suspected. She would try eating the low-carbohydrate, high-protein, frequent-small-feeding diet that one friend had recommended so highly. She went home eager to try her new cure.

Although Doris's doctor wasn't deliberately lying, he had made a grave error by letting his patient pressure him into giving her a "name." Hypoglycemia—like anemia—is not an actual disease; it is simply a phenomenon that indicates any one of many diseases. Patients with hypoglycemia have blood glucose levels too low to meet the immediate energy needs of their body tissues. To know whether a patient has hypoglycemia, then, a doctor merely has to run a test of the patient's blood sugar level at the same time that she is feeling unenergetic.[4] But because Doris's doctor didn't want to disappoint his patient, he substituted a probable description for a disease, and Doris went home thinking that all her problems had been solved.

This kind of behavior is not only misguided; it can keep people from the treatment they need. In his book on hypoglycemia, Dr. Lynn Bennon describes a patient, Mr. Engelhardt, who had hypoglycemia; his blood glucose was too low to meet his needs. Unlike Doris's doctor, however, Dr. Bennon did not consider "hypoglycemia" a sufficient diagnosis because Mr. Engelhardt's *disease* was not hypoglycemia. Rather, hypoglycemia was merely a clue to his actual disease: adrenal-gland failure. According to Dr. Bennon, Mr. Engelhardt's supply of adrenal-gland hormones was now cut off. "For treatment [he] needed replacement of those missing adrenal hormones, either by injection or by pills," notes Dr. Bennon.[5] Clearly, in Mr. Engelhardt's case, it was not enough to know that he had "hypoglycemia" if he was to get effective treatment, for Doris's diet would not help restore his hormone levels.

Similarly, adds Dr. Bennon, people who regard anemia as a disease may try to raise their hemoglobin levels by taking liver and iron pills. This might make sense if anemia were a disease caused by low hemoglobin levels: by raising the hemoglobin levels, the symptoms of this "disease," anemia, might disappear. But, again, anemia is not a disease. As Dr. Bennon points out, "If someone is anemic, there is something wrong that is causing the hemoglobin level to be low. The intelligent first step is to figure out *why* the person has anemia. Malaria might be the cause of the anemia, or hookworms in the intestine, or a bleeding ulcer, or a cancer of the rectum. Or in a child it might be lead poisoning from chewing on lead paint on the windowsill."[6] Clearly, a few iron pills are not going to help cure these serious conditions; no matter how many pills the patient takes, he will continue to have anemia until someone takes care of his underlying disease.

▲ TAKING MORE THAN YOUR SHARE

A third way that people confuse symptoms with diseases is evident when people start acting as though having a symptom of a disease were the same thing as having the disease itself. Confusion results because one symptom can be shared by many different diseases; thus, if you have an epileptic seizure, a symptom of the disease epilepsy, you don't necessarily have epilepsy. One seizure, though identical to the seizure of an epileptic, may result from inhaling noxious fumes; only someone with *recurrent* epileptic seizures has the disease.[7]

Symptoms associated with more than one disease can underlie years of misdiagnosis. Consider my maternal uncle, who for decades has been trying different diets to soothe his nausea and other gastrointestinal distress, which doctors for years suggested could be caused by food allergies. One time when I visited my uncle, he couldn't eat anything with gluten in it. The next time I saw him, he couldn't eat meat. At other times, he was avoiding chicken livers, MSG, and chocolate. No diet seemed to help sufficiently, however, nor did any of the medications he took or the surgical procedures he underwent (treatments that themselves were sometimes cited as the source of his complaints). At one point he was diagnosed and treated for Crohn's disease (regional ileitis), a condition of unknown origin which involves inflammation of part of the small intestine and which is sometimes (incorrectly) assumed to be of psychological origin.

At one point, too, my uncle started to sense his blood pressure rising. "I found myself babbling and watching myself babbling, trying to say something and finding something else come out of my mouth," he recalls. "I also had some psychological symptoms—depression and wanting to be alone when I felt that way." At last all these symptoms seemed to overpower him, and he ended up being rushed to the hospital in an ambulance. "They did all sorts of tests—brain scans, heart monitors—but no one had any idea what was wrong with me. When I came back to my hometown, however, my doctor knew right away what I had, because she shared the same problem: migraine."

Migraines, or migraine headaches, which afflict at least forty-one out of every thousand Americans, can be considered a nameless disease.[8] Involving much more than severe recurrent headaches, migraines are a whole complex or pattern of symptoms that can include numbness, prickling, tingling, nausea, vomiting, light sensitivity, depression, and irritability—and, indeed, need not even involve a headache to be classified as "migraine equivalents." "Classic migraine" also involves an aura or premonition of the migraine to come, the symptoms of which can include visual and other sensory hallucinations, mosaic vision, "doubling of consciousness" (e.g., déjà vu), gradual loss of consciousness, disorders of thinking and language, mood changes, and transient weakness in arms or legs. Clearly many of these symptoms are shared by other conditions, and by focusing on my uncle's gastrointestinal problems rather than on the whole range of symptoms, doctors for years had missed diagnosing migraine, a condition that my uncle now believes accounts for many of his past health problems and psychological troubles.

"Once I had this name, I realized that I had had migraines all my life but had always associated them with these terrible GI [gastrointestinal] symptoms and not really noticed the headache part at all," he says. "After we fixed up the GI troubles, only then did I notice the headache symptoms more. Looking at the list of foods that supposedly aggravated migraines, I also realized that these were all foods that at one point or another I had cut out of my life to alleviate other symptoms. . . . But fixing up the GI meant a lot of medication, dietary changes, and even surgery, that I might not have needed had I known it was migraine all along—which is better treated with psychotherapy."

Shared symptoms can also plague the diagnosis of women who think they may suffer from premenstrual syndrome. This syndrome is characterized by a wide range of symptoms, including migraines, epilepsy, depression, eating disorders, irrational rages, and alcoholism, and (as noted in Chapter 2) their specific nature isn't as important as their timing. So long as the symptoms, whatever they may be, occur at the same time each month, a woman may be suffering from PMS. What this means is that a woman with PMS *may* suffer from headaches or eating binges or temper tantrums; but that does not mean that anyone suffering from headaches, eating binges, or temper tantrums necessarily has PMS.

All this may seem obvious, but there are plenty of women who snap at their three-year-olds one day and go around saying that they have PMS the next. Even so-called authorities on PMS frequently confuse symptoms with the disease. In several popular books on PMS, the authors make an unconscious leap of faith—equating a woman's depression with PMS, for example, without looking into the woman's menstrual history or trying to correlate this depression with the premenstrual days. Thus, one book ostensibly on PMS ends up being a chronicle of all stages of a female's life and health, with or without PMS—since there are very few women who go through life without *ever* feeling depressed, overeating, or having a headache.[9]

This can be carried to ludicrous extremes. In another book on PMS, the authors describe a medical researcher who was investigating the effects of the hormone prolactin, which, among other things, stimulates the mammary glands.[10] When he injected himself with this hormone, his body swelled up and he felt irritable and "fed up with it all." The authors then write that today this researcher says his experiences "were remarkably like those of women having premenstrual syndrome. He suggests, only half humorously, that he may be the only male in history to have been 'premenstrual.'"[11]

It is clear from this example that symptoms are not necessarily unique to one specific disease. Feeling "fed up" or having "swollen tissues" are not just the symptoms of PMS (obviously this male researcher did not have PMS); they can be the result of excess prolactin. Nor does this research mean that all women with PMS have excess prolactin levels: there are many reasons, after all, why we could feel "fed up."[12]

Another book, this one on puerperal mental illness, extends definitions just as generously. Even though the early chapters explain how the postpartum depression (PPD) probably results from hormonal changes that take place in women after childbirth and deserves disease status, later chapters discuss the multitude of people who may suffer PPD—people including adoptive mothers and, yes, even fathers![13] Suddenly, anyone who experiences depression or moodiness within a few days, weeks, or even years after a new arrival can share in the title "PPD."

Undoubtedly, the desire to sell popular medical books fuels such errors of logic: after all, the more people who can relate to a book's topic, the more copies will sell. One particularly blatant example is a book entitled *Chronic Fatigue Syndrome: The Hidden Epidemic.* Chronic fatigue syndrome (also known as chronic fatigue immune dysfunction syndrome, or CFIDS) has been an officially recognized syndrome (though still poorly defined) by the Centers for Disease Control in Atlanta, Georgia, since May 1988, and if the book really addressed that syndrome, then the title would be legitimate. But the book instead turns out to be about an idiosyncratic, holistic, homeopathic approach to healing, with special reference to something called "chronic Epstein-Barr virus disease," which the authors (incorrectly) equate with chronic fatigue syndrome early in the book. Thereafter, the authors drop the term "chronic fatigue syndrome" entirely and talk about stress, visualization, and nutritional healing. It seems that the only reason they use the term "fatigue" in the title is to entice all the people who feel fatigued most of the time (and 25 percent of Americans believe that they do!).[14]

Behavioral conditions are even more vulnerable to this kind of abuse. One author, for example, describes a little boy who is having trouble in school. She asks: "Is Billy simply 'immature,' or does he have a 'learning disability?'"[15] Her question implies that if Billy has the latter "disease," he is somehow relieved of the embarrassing immaturity. It is not accidental that the author writes "learning disability" rather than "learns with difficulty," or "immature" rather than "acts younger than his age." By writing of specific attributes that Billy might have (immaturity or a learning disability) rather than Billy's actions (learns with difficulty and acts immaturely), the author offers a choice between one of two names—"immature" or "learning disabled"—each with its own set of associations.

As it turns out, it is better to have the name "learning disabled" than it is to have the name "immature," just as it is better to have "PMS" than it is to be "moody" or "crazy." And it's easy to pick and choose among symptoms and disease names. Many social problems accompany learning disabilities; therefore, just about *any* social problem—including poor conversation skills, rudeness, laziness, or selfishness—may be attributed to a learning disability, even though these problems can have many other causes. If you examine the statements of many advocates of "learning disability" as a specific disease, in fact, it begins to look as though anyone, with any sort of adjustment problem, is "learning disabled."[16]

Because it is so easy to be defined as having a disease (all you need is one of the symptoms), it's no wonder that people often claim to have many of the more poorly defined, new diseases. Thus, one doctor at a PMS meeting contended that PMS may be an adult form of hyperactivity (which many equate with dyslexia or learning disabilities). In fact, Dr. Katharina Dalton, a leading authority on premenstrual syndrome, claimed that she has suffered not only from PMS but from dyslexia as well. Many of her peers agreed: learning disorders and PMS may be correlated. Then another doctor linked PMS with puerperal mental illness. He remembered a time when he was a police surgeon in an area north of London. He was called out one night to see a woman "behaving strangely." At one in the morning she was lying in the middle of a busy street with her two children, speaking gibberish. Her husband complained, "God, every time she has a bleeding baby, she does this." Now, since meeting this couple, the doctor always suspects PMS in women with puerperal depression. All of these correlations may, of course, prove true in the end, but at the moment they just jumble up already confusing studies: just behaving hyperactively is not the same as having dyslexia; just behaving irrationally is not the same as having PMS.

▲ KEEPING SYMPTOMS AND DISEASES STRAIGHT

The obvious solution to this confusion, of course, would be to distinguish carefully the meaning of "symptom" from the meaning of "disease." And, in fact, any medical dictionary will tell you what a symptom is. One, for example, defines a symptom as "any subjective evidence of disease or of a patient's condition, i.e., such evidence as perceived by the patient; a change in a patient's condition indicative of some bodily or mental state."[17] On the surface, that sounds straightforward enough. On closer inspection, though, the distinction is not so simple.

First of all, some diseases have no symptoms at all. The disease "hypertension," for example, is defined as elevated blood pressure; blood pressure can rise for a number of reasons, and people with hypertension are at great risk of developing several very serious illnesses. But there are no symptoms of hypertension itself—not even the blood pressure reading—because this is something that a doctor measures, not something that a patient perceives; it is not a symptom.[18] Some people with hypertension may argue this point and claim that they can feel it when their blood pressure rises, but many studies have shown that hypertensives who believe they can detect their own blood pressure are usually wrong; so are people who believe that their blood pressure is higher when they feel tense or angry. In fact, because hypertension has no symptoms, doctors have trouble persuading undiagnosed hypertensives to begin treatment and even more trouble keeping patients on their medications: the patients feel fine, after all. To control this "silent killer," investigators are trying to identify some other symptoms, but attempts so far have been unsuccessful.[19]

Complicating matters further, symptoms can themselves have symptoms. Fainting, for example, can have many symptoms of its own, including weakness, giddiness, distorted vision, sweating, nausea, and vomiting. Similarly, the symptoms of indigestion can include belching, abdominal distention, lack of appetite, and nausea. I am not playing word games here: if you look in any standard medical text, you will see fainting ("syncope") and indigestion ("dyspepsia") listed as symptoms under many different diseases; but if you then look up fainting and indigestion, you will see a long list of their symptoms as well. Suddenly the dictionary definitions start to look inadequate.

All that's well and good, you may be thinking, but most of the time I can tell a symptom from a disease. Maybe the man in the street can't give you a rock-hard definition, but he certainly knows intuitively that fever is the symptom and flu is the disease.

Or can he? I'll grant you that a late-twentieth-century person can tell you the relationship between fever and flu. But if you went back in time and asked the average person the same question, he would answer differently. To the eighteenth-century man in the street, for example, "fever" was more than a shorthand term for high body temperature: it was a disease or pattern in its own right, and it had its own explanation, its own set of symptoms, perhaps even its own treatment. Hearing the word "fever," an eighteenth-century person would not think much—if anything—about exact body temperature (doctors rarely used thermometers before the mid-1800s); instead, one might think about someone with a quick pulse rate, increased body temperature, chills, and overall weakness.[20] In other words, fever was not just one feature of many diseases but was itself a pattern composed of many features—just as we now think of flu or measles as a pattern of many features, one of which may be a fever.

Eighteenth-century doctors actually talked about many kinds of fevers: "hectic fever," "intermittent fever," "bilious fever," "ague and fever," "acute continual fever," "relapsing fever," and others. These terms referred to various characteristics of the fever: how stable were the symptoms, how often did they recur, what were their causes, and so on. "Acute continual fever," for example, meant a relatively short and steady but violent disease. This is how Dr. William Buchan, a popular writer, described it to his lay readers in 1772:

> A rigour or chillness generally ushers in this fever, which is soon succeeded by great heat, a frequent and full pulse, a pain of the head, dry skin, redness of the eyes, a florid countenance, pains in the back, loins, etc. To these succeed difficulty of breathing, sickness, with an inclina-

tion to vomit. The patient complains of great thirst, has no
appetite for solid food, is restless, and his tongue generally appears black or rough.

Very sick patients might also become delirious, with "laborious
respiration, straining of the tendons, hiccup, cold, clammy sweats, and
an involuntary discharge of urine."[21] Modern doctors might have said
that the patients described here had any one of many diseases and that
a black tongue or difficult breathing were symptoms of that disease,
just as the fever was. For Buchan, though, everything he saw added up
into one pattern: acute, continual fever.

As doctors gained more experience with sick patients, they had
to recategorize some of the fevers they had described earlier. In fact, by
the time Dr. Gunn described fever to his readers of 1830, he sometimes
used "fever" to mean a symptom, as we do today; fever could be a
symptom of either inflammatory rheumatism or inflammation of the
spleen, for example.[22] At other times, however, Gunn called fever a
"disease," although, as noted above in Chapter 3, he used the term "disease" rather loosely, often meaning a vague dis-ease (i.e., discomfort)
rather than a specific pattern. Like many of his predecessors (and some
of his successors), in fact, Gunn never developed even an internally
consistent way to use such terms as "symptom" and "disease," so it's
not completely clear whether he really considered "fever" to be a disease in the sense we call measles a disease.[23]

But there is no doubt that Dr. Gunn, like many eighteenth-
century doctors before him, and like many other practitioners of the
day who were still unfamiliar with the work going on in elite medical
circles, still described certain forms of fever as if they were very distinct
diseases, each with its own set of causes, symptoms, and treatments.
The disease "ague and fever," for example, had three stages—the
"cold," the "hot," and the "sweating." The first comes on every twenty-
four hours, the second every forty, and the third every forty-eight.[24] And
the symptoms of the *very dangerous* disease "nervous (or typhus)
fever" were

a constant inclination to throw off the cover; a changing of
the voice from its usual tone; great vigilance or watch-
fulness; picking at the bed-clothing; inability to hold or
retain the urine; involuntary discharges from the bowels;
hiccuping; a muttering as if speaking to one's self; a wild

and fixed look, as if the eyes were rivetted [sic] on some
particular object.[25]

If you think about how it feels to lie in bed with a temperature of
102 degrees, you will begin to understand how someone could interpret "picking at the bed-clothing" as a symptom of a disease. Imagine
now that a doctor, innocent of modern medical ideas, comes to see
you. Lying there sweltering, you may very well kick off the covers. You
almost certainly will sweat a great deal, and if this fictive doctor feels
like measuring your pulse, he may well find that it's a little quicker than
he expects. Aching and miserable, you may stare straight ahead. After
seeing many patients lying in bed and acting this way, a doctor without
preconceived notions about what to notice may very well say: "I see
many patients who lie in bed sweating, with rapid pulses and fixed
stares, who kick off the bedcovers. All of these symptoms are part of
the disease 'fever.'"

Of course, you, with all your modern notions, know that you
"really" have the flu, and having the flu doesn't mean you're necessarily
going to kick off the bedcovers. But, again, even if you don't happen to
do this, our innocent doctor has a way out: nobody shows all the symptoms of any disease (not everyone with a cold has laryngitis, after all),
but you still show enough to have fever. What if you don't sweat either,
and your pulse is even a bit slow? Well, if too many things don't fit, the
doctor might just say you have a different kind of fever—maybe "ague
and fever" or "bilious fever." He has seen patients before just like you.

Nor would he be a raving idiot: there is no doubt that many earlier doctors truly "saw" in their patients all the features of fever that they
described. Furthermore, with several notable exceptions, patients in
the eighteenth and nineteenth century probably were not suffering
from anything very different from what patients suffer from today. In
fact, if we took a feverish eighteenth-century man through a time machine and stuck a thermometer in his mouth, we'd probably find that
his temperature was higher than 98.6 degrees. The only difference is
that earlier doctors had a different idea of relevant characteristics to
lump together and call a disease.

In other words, when modern doctors see features like sweating
or "disturbed circulation," they don't see them as symptoms of a larger
pattern, but as basically irrelevant by-products of an elevated temperature. Instead of relying on these features to distinguish one condition
from the next, today's doctors rely on observations afforded by better

technology: they consider the microorganism or the internal lesion or the incubation period associated with that fever as significant ways to divide patients, not whether they have high temperatures. Only someone with preconceptions about which events are relevant, however, can be expected to realize that what matters is not your relationship with your sheets but whether or not you have a flu virus in your blood.

So then, what is it about this pattern called the flu that makes us realize it is different from the thing we call a symptom (when, in other cultures, the thing we call a symptom might appear to be a pattern, a disease)? Medical dictionaries talk in circles, defining symptoms in terms of diseases and diseases in terms of symptoms. Just as there is no single criterion used to separate one disease from another, there is no single criterion used to separate a symptom from a disease. Intuitively, of course, we usually can distinguish the disease—the flu— from the symptoms—the fever and the aching. We usually think that the things we "feel" or "measure" are the symptoms; we must "derive" the disease through logic. The symptoms are real, immediately obvious, but the disease is abstract, something we have to "figure out." Some would add that this disease is what causes the symptoms. But these intuitions, once we try to get beyond a few obvious examples from our everyday lives, are not always helpful. As we have seen, what we regard as symptoms may themselves, in other times or places, be regarded as diseases; that is, other cultures may consider what we regard as a concrete, observable event to represent a coherent pattern of several other concrete, observable events. Furthermore, since diseases are merely patterns—abstract groupings of phenomena—it doesn't make sense to say that diseases "cause" symptoms; patterns aren't capable of causing anything.

The best we can do to keep diseases and symptoms straight is to recognize that a disease is a mutually acknowledged pattern; that this pattern is not hard-and-fast, but can change in different times and places; and that, above all, this pattern is assumed within any given culture to have a unique cause, even if we don't happen to know that cause at present. In contrast, a symptom, which can itself be a pattern of other symptoms (a symptom-complex), is not assumed to have a unique cause; it is a sort of small, subordinate, nonspecific pattern that can be part of many different disease patterns and, unlike a disease pattern, can result from many different causes.[26]

My grandmother, then, had a lot in common with some renowned ancient physicians: she interpreted something we regard as a symptom to be a disease. Like fever, headache, toothache, sore throat, rheumatism, arthritis, asthma, and severe shock ("congestive fever"), many nonunique conditions were once regarded as complete, unique, and specific diseases by earlier physicians. In fact, as we shall see, even today laymen sometimes use names (such as rheumatism) in their old sense to mean a disease while doctors use them in the modern sense to mean a symptom.[27]

Furthermore, the same term can be viewed as a disease in one context and as a symptom in another. A dictionary definition is not going to help separate these two points of view. Such definitions make a lot of sense if you share a certain core of knowledge—that is, if you know what the doctors of your time consider to be uniquely determined diseases—but if you're starting from scratch, it's easy enough to confuse a symptom with a disease. If no one has told you the relevant patterns and features to begin with, it's pretty easy to find symptoms in almost anything (Dr. Gunn's "throwing off the bedcovers" as a symptom of "nervous fever") and regard the entire complex of symptoms as a uniquely determined pattern. Couple that with the enormous relief which comes from having a disease name attached to your discomfort, and you'll begin to understand why it's so easy to take almost any name assigned to a condition and immediately assume that the name stands for a full-fledged disease.

CHAPTER 6

▲

Mistaking Syndromes for Diseases

It seems that every time I open a newspaper there's a new syndrome: premenstrual syndrome, Tourette syndrome, acquired immunodeficiency syndrome, Reye's syndrome, sudden infant death syndrome, Rett syndrome, fetal alcohol syndrome, holiday depression syndrome, delayed pregnancy syndrome, and even the unmade-bed syndrome, the Peter Pan syndrome, the good girl syndrome, the battered wife syndrome, and the adopted child syndrome. Naming a new syndrome can mean a quick path to fame and fortune. Many new syndromes are promoted by support groups that churn out press releases and provide fodder for bestselling books and television talk shows, not to mention successful legal defenses. It's no wonder, then, that I sometimes feel there's a "syndrome of the week." This week alone I saw Tourette syndrome described in an Ann Landers column, a *People* magazine feature, and a *Boston Globe* article.

Not that there is anything inherently wrong in naming a new syndrome. Syndromes can represent a legitimate medical category, especially useful for conditions that are more than just symptoms but not really full diseases. A syndrome (or symptom-complex) is a recurring and as yet unexplained collection of signs and symptoms, one not yet linked to a unique and specific cause, even hypothetically. Let's say that certain blondes tend to develop big red spots on their left cheeks and get uncontrollable hiccups after eating chocolate ice cream; when they eat whipped cream along with the ice cream, however, the symptoms quickly subside. A doctor who notices all this may call the problem "chocolate ice cream syndrome," and the next time he sees a blonde woman with a red blotch on her cheek, empty Dixie cup in hand and hiccuping away, he can quickly administer a dose of whipped cream. Note that if he hadn't known about chocolate ice cream syndrome, he might have told the ailing woman that she needed a horror movie for her hiccups and a good cover-up cream for her face. Knowing about it, however, he is able to prescribe a quick remedy (whipped cream). Calling something a syndrome, therefore, is a particularly useful way to describe conditions about which we still know very little.

Utility notwithstanding, a syndrome is not the same thing as a disease. Sometimes, later knowledge will show that a given syndrome can be produced only when many diseases appear together. Chocolate ice cream syndrome, for example, may result only when people have a sun allergy, a metabolic disorder, and a congenitally narrow throat— but when people have only one of these diseases, they experience no problems from eating chocolate ice cream. On the other hand, a syndrome may result when someone has any one of several different diseases; thus, chocolate ice cream syndrome may appear in certain types of psychoses, among blondes with bronchitis, or even after peroxide poisoning. It may even turn out that a syndrome is associated with just one disease: perhaps chocolate ice cream syndrome results only after an infection by the as yet undiscovered "chocovirus," which has a preference for blondes. Only then would it be legitimate to regard this syndrome as a full-fledged disease.

At this point, however, no one really knows which—if any—of these explanations is true. And it doesn't matter. So long as something is called a "syndrome," doctors are openly admitting that they're not quite sure whether this state is linked with one or with many diseases. All that matters is that the group of signs and symptoms (e.g., blondeness, hiccuping, red spots, chocolate ice cream, and whipped cream) are associated, not what produces them. Nobody is making any claim yet about whether there are one or more explanations or types of this syndrome.

In contrast, when doctors call something a disease they are implying that they know a little more, at least enough to assume—even if it hasn't been proven yet—that this condition represents one kind of pattern.[1] At least they are implying this in theory, and that's where the problems with syndromes begin. In practice, most people (including most doctors) use the terms "disease" and "syndrome" rather loosely; for example, while some gynecologists would say that a hairy, obese woman who doesn't menstruate has "polycystic ovary *syndrome*," others would say she has "polycystic ovary *disease*." Even the same writer will often fling these terms around, carefully defining syndrome on one page and then, several pages later, using the words "disease" and "syndrome" synonymously. Others may explain that conditions like AIDS, endometriosis, or epilepsy are not diseases, but then proceed to talk about them as if each were a single entity, each with a common and specific origin and outcome.[2]

A few years ago, for example, my local newspaper's science section featured an article on the "chronic mono syndrome"—now known as chronic fatigue immune dysfunction syndrome (CFIDS) or chronic fatigue syndrome since investigators have determined that the Epstein-Barr virus, known to cause mononucleosis, is not the exclusive or principal cause of this new syndrome.[3] CFIDS is apparently a new condition: doctors noticed the first cases in late 1984, although retrospective studies suggest that some people developed the syndrome as long ago as 1979. The victims—most commonly affluent, well-educated women, especially in California and Nevada—experience a disabling fatigue that lasts at least six months; they also develop persistent sore throats, swollen lymph glands, fevers, muscle aches, and weakness. Other symptoms can include night sweats, severe headaches, confusion, memory problems, disturbed balance, depression, sleep disorders, anxiety, prickling sensations, visual disturbances, involuntary muscle contractions, ringing in the ears, recurrent respiratory infections, allergies, urinary tract infections, mouth ulcers, chest and abdominal pain, nausea, breathing problems, heart palpitations, and inflammation of the heart muscle. Patients take years to recover, or don't seem to recover at all, and so far doctors know no definite cause.

All this sounds very much like a syndrome—a collection of associated symptoms and signs—and yet the article describes "chronic mono syndrome" as both a "syndrome" and a "disease." Throughout, in fact, the terms are used interchangeably, even in the headline: "The Baffling 'Chronic Mono' *Syndrome:* The *disease, a collection of symptoms,* can disable its victims with fatigue and prolonged flu-like illness" (emphasis added). Later the article's author, Richard A. Knox, points out that this "disease" is extremely difficult to define precisely, since the symptoms mimic many common disorders, and there is no diagnostic laboratory test that can pin it down. Learning the name "chronic mono syndrome" should be a boon to many patients, he adds, because many doctors may hitherto have called these patients mentally ill, owing to a deep bias in the medical profession against vague, hard-to-diagnose "diseases" such as "fatigue." Knox cites Dr. James Jones, of National Jewish Hospital, who received a $300,000 federal grant to study the syndrome; according to Knox, Dr. Jones says that this prejudice against hard-to-diagnose "diseases" has caused "untold anguish to patients suffering from the syndrome. They often bounce from one doctor to another, convinced either that something is terribly, organically wrong—or that they're 'going crazy.'"[4]

All of this makes CFIDS sound very much like a nameless disease, which indeed we have called it earlier. Just like people with nameless diseases, victims of this syndrome—as with so many newly named syndromes—may bounce from doctor to doctor, never learning the name of their condition. They may think that they are "crazy" or "evil" or "hypochondriacal," especially because there is no clear-cut laboratory test that can reveal a biological marker for their condition. And when sufferers find out that they do have one of these new syndromes, they feel tremendous relief. In short, finding out that you have one of these new syndromes is a lot like finding out that you have a nameless disease. In fact, many of the conditions I've called "nameless diseases" are syndromes—for example, premenstrual syndrome and Rett syndrome—because the medical community as a whole still hasn't decided whether or not they represent one unified pattern. Not enough is yet known about syndromes or nameless diseases to regard them as monolithic disease entities.

What is crucial to understand here is that so-called syndromes (and the many "nameless diseases" that remain syndromes, whatever their names) are not full-fledged diseases. As we saw with the hypothetical "chocolate ice cream syndrome," the same syndrome can have many different causes, and people with the same syndrome can have very different diseases. When doctors tell you that you have a syndrome, they are implying that although you share certain characteristics with other patients and although what is true for them might be true for you, you might *also* have some entirely different disease. At this point, the doctors still don't quite know. Consequently, although you may be relieved to find a name for your syndrome, confusing this name with a disease is a way of getting all the benefits of a name without any of the responsibilities.

▲ REAPING THE BENEFITS

People confuse syndromes with diseases for the same reason they confuse symptoms with diseases: the benefits of having a recognized disease are too tempting to ignore. A name provides relief from anxiety and guilt, and it often provides a ready-made social and medical network, as well.

It's this kind of thinking that allows reporters to dash off a list of famous people who may have suffered from "manic depression."[5] This condition is more like a syndrome than a disease: psychiatrists still don't know if the symptoms and signs are part of one entity or many. But the same journalists who acknowledge this uncertainty were still quick to assume that one gene caused manic depression when researchers found that a gene might be responsible for manic-depressive behavior in several Amish families. They never paused to consider that this particular manic-depressive behavior might be one of several forms and that the gene in the Amish families might have nothing to do with the manic-depressive behavior seen in other people. By way of forging more positive connotations, moreover (see Chapter 1, above, on "in" diseases), these journalists were equally quick to cite all the talented people who may have suffered from "manic depression," including the composers George Frideric Handel and Gustav Mahler, the poets Robert Lowell, John Berryman, and Anne Sexton, the statesmen Theodore Roosevelt and Winston Churchill (who also gets cited by the dyslexia people), as well as numerous artists and financial wizards. Even though all these people might have suffered from a variety of diseases which produced manic-depressive symptoms, there was absolutely no new evidence that these people carried the same gene as the Amish families. Even so, it is often handy to lump all people with symptoms of manic depression together in order to make a rhetorical point.

In the same way, a chapter in a well-known medical textbook notes that "gout" is not one disease but a heterogeneous group of genetic and acquired diseases that share similar signs and symptoms. And yet, despite this pronouncement, the rest of the chapter treats gout not as a syndrome, but as an "it" that has afflicted mankind for more than twenty-five hundred years; it also cites notable victims including Alexander the Great, Queen Anne, Francis Bacon, John Calvin, Charlemagne, Charles Darwin, Leonardo da Vinci, Benjamin Franklin, Goethe, Henry VIII, Samuel Johnson, Louis XIV, Martin Luther, John Milton, Isaac Newton, and both the elder and the younger William Pitt.[6]

As we saw in Chapter 1, similar sleights of hand occur with PMS and dyslexia, which, given current data, are more syndromes than they are full-fledged diseases. Whether or not it turns out that these conditions reflect one specific disease, many advocates of their disease status stretch the available data to extremes in order to name an otherwise unjustifiable behavior. One popular book on PMS, for example, says quite clearly that the term PMS may include many different types of patients and that a woman with nausea and breast-bloating before her period may not have the same disease as a woman with monthly desires to bludgeon her husband. Nevertheless, throughout the rest of the book the authors frequently assume that anyone with any of a hundred or so symptoms has this thing called "PMS"; they never distinguish between one type of PMS and another.[7] In fact, the authors actually suggest that PMS underlay the Lizzie Borden axe murders. Granted, they never argue that such behavior is justified, PMS or no PMS, and they stress that PMS did not cause these crimes. But the fact remains: we feel more sympathy toward Lizzie if we think of her as a victim of PMS, a specific disease with a probable hormonal base, than if we think of her as an evil woman. In the same way, a man may prefer to think that his wife occasionally calls him unprintable names, throws wine in his face, slaps up the toddler, and smashes the fender because of PMS.

The broad definition of PMS, as with most of the nameless diseases, makes it quite easy to assign the label liberally. After all, PMS can appear fifteen days out of every thirty, and there are hundreds of symptoms to choose from, many of which are "moods." All that's required for any of these symptoms to be diagnosed as part of PMS is that it recur monthly.[8] Now, how many women really record whether every single irrational act and bad mood occurred in the same half (in relation to the menstrual period) of each month? Isn't it rather likely that, if you want to, you can decide that you definitely feel moodier during the fifteen days before your period rather than the fifteen days after? Isn't it tempting, then, to cite PMS as the culprit for an otherwise irreconcilable marriage, living situation, or personality?

Not only is it tempting, but it happens frequently. According to several studies, in fact, 50 percent of women self-diagnosed as having PMS actually have other forms of psychiatric problems.[9] Furthermore, broad names also lead to blurring one condition with the next. Many investigators have noticed, for example, that women labeled as having puerperal mental illness and women labeled as having PMS often have many common symptoms.[10] These include fatigue, depression, irritability, increased thirst and appetite, headaches, breast-swelling and abdominal bloating, swollen extremities, constipation, and acne. True, both of these nameless diseases seem related to reproductive hormones, but at present such broad symptoms make these terms so loose that they cease to have much meaning.

Please recognize that I am not denying that PMS is a serious and very real problem for some women; I am merely explaining why the term is abused and misapplied to many others. We all want excuses for anything negative in our character or behavior, and, indeed, there is nearly always some explanation for justifying undesirable events; few, if any, people are just plain "evil." But whether it's helpful to name these broad explanations, these broad syndromes, as diseases and focus on them that way—that's the question.

As it turns out, latching onto such labels for nameless diseases may spread the benefits of a name too thin: to call just about everything "PMS" will soon make having "PMS" irrelevant. Indiscriminate labeling quickly reaches the point of absurdity, so that genuine sufferers aren't taken seriously. Specifically, women who snap at their husbands one day and say "Oh, it's my PMS" make laughingstocks of the true sufferers.[11]

▲ BEARING THE BURDENS

Perhaps because syndromes are by definition looser terms than diseases, many professionals tend to invent them rather irresponsibly. In particular, these "pseudosyndromes," as one writer has called them, can cause unanticipated anguish for people who are unwittingly linked with others by virtue of sharing the same condition. For example, an article in the October 1986 issue of *Ms.* by Francine Klagsbrun debunks what had been called the "adopted child syndrome." Apparently this term was first used by a defense psychologist in the trial of an adopted teenager accused of setting fire to his home and murdering his parents. According to the psychologist, the young man's behavior was "a classic example of a syndrome that included such traits as preoccupation with excessive fantasy, setting fires, learning difficulties, lack of impulse control, pathological lying, theft, defiance of authority, and running away from home." However, since the term was unproven and unrecognized in psychiatric manuals, the boy was found guilty of second-degree murder and arson.

Next, reports Klagsbrun, an article by Betty Jean Lifton (a well-known activist for change in the adoption system) appeared on the op-ed page of the *New York Times.* Not only does Klagsbrun say that Lifton concurred with the psychologist's terminology, she says that Lifton extended it: "'most adoptees,' Lifton wrote, "exhibit some of these traits as a result of their confusion about heritage.'" Lifton proceeded to list the names of many vicious killers who had been adopted and, according to Klagsbrun, "implied that unless adoption records are unsealed and adoptees given access to extensive information about their origins, society is likely to be terrorized by continued violence from frustrated adoptees."

Klagsbrun, a writer on social issues who happened to be an adoptive parent as well, did not appreciate that the use of a name, "adopted child syndrome," helped diminish the guilt possibly felt by all these vicious killers. Rather, she thought of her own nonviolent children and was quite disturbed at their instant stigmatization. She searched through the scientific literature but could find no mention of the term "adopted child syndrome." Nor could she find much evidence of anything particularly abnormal in adopted children, except perhaps an overrepresentation in psychiatric treatment. So she called up the psychologist who had used the term in court, and lo and behold he acknowledged—proudly, writes Klagsbrun—that he had coined the term himself. She writes: "He had disseminated some written information on his syndrome through his own clinic in Merrick, Long Island, but no, he had published nothing on it in recognized psychiatric journals. He estimates that about 10 percent of the adopted population exhibit symptoms of the syndrome, but no, he has gathered no hard-and-fast data to support that." The psychologist thought that the syndrome seemed to appear with children who had had difficult adoptions (e.g., repeated separations from foster parents and parents or adoption at older ages), but he had not statistically drawn distinctions between these children and other adoptees. Klagsbrun concludes: "So there it is. An unsubstantiated 'disease' classification is used to buttress the defense in a criminal case, then irresponsibly misused to prove a point, and suddenly all adopted children and their parents find themselves somehow tainted and stigmatized." [12]

▲ FATAL CONSEQUENCES

The other night I happened upon a television show about a forty-four-year-old woman whose nine children, one after another, had died as infants or toddlers, all except the first of unexplained natural causes, or sudden infant death syndrome (SIDS). According to the *Merck Manual,* SIDS is simply "the unexpected and unexplained death of an apparently well, or virtually well, infant." In other words, parents tuck their baby in for the night and return several hours later to find it dead. The cause is entirely unknown, although doctors suspect that SIDS might be related to a breathing problem brought on by any one of many conditions. Although the most frequent victims are babies three to four months old, SIDS is the most common cause of death for all infants worldwide between the ages of two weeks and one year. In fact, between 8,000 and 10,000 infants die from SIDS in the United States every year.[13]

To lose just one baby to SIDS would be devastating for any parent; for this woman to have lost so many seemed unfathomable. It also seemed bizarre: SIDS appears to strike randomly, but this family story suggested that SIDS was somehow hereditary. Although the woman's doctors couldn't find any research supporting this theory, they had encouraged her to adopt after she lost several children. And yet, the adopted baby also died of SIDS. Was this woman just cursed, then, or was there perhaps something lethal to babies in the home environment?

After much investigation, it turned out that there *was* something lethal in the home: the mother herself. Investigators at last began to suspect that she had strangled each of her children, one by one.[14] When the coroner examined these infants, he noted that each had died from suffocation for no known reason, and he duly recorded "SIDS." Although literally accurate, assigning that label had been a fatal mistake. If the death certificate had simply read "suffocation for no clear reason" or "unknown cause of death," it is quite likely that someone along the way would have suspected foul play after just one child had been killed. Instead, though, doctors, relatives, even law enforcement officials all saw the name of a disease and simply assumed that the medical community must not know very much about this "disease." As a result, nine babies had to die.

All of this was quite upsetting to the National Sudden Infant Death Syndrome Foundation. They were concerned that this woman's story would encourage the public to attach the stigma of "murderer" to any parent who lost a baby. For years before anyone talked about SIDS, in fact, parents whose babies died spontaneously were indeed subject to all sorts of accusations and feelings of guilt. Because they were not prepared for such a tragedy, they were especially vulnerable in the face of investigations conducted by police and social workers and even the questions of sympathetic friends. Thus, the name "SIDS" helped assure these parents that their baby had died of a real "disease." However humane this position, it nonetheless ignores the reality that there is still no evidence that SIDS is a single disease entity; it is merely a syndrome, a catchall term for spontaneous infant death that can have any one of many causes, only some of which deserve every ounce of sympathy and support a foundation can muster. Often the cause might be spontaneous lung failure; sometimes it might be a respiratory infection; and rarely, but only rarely, it may turn out to be murder.

▲ CATCHALL TERMS

The consequences of confusing syndromes with diseases, then, can be extremely severe. Unfortunately, too, those conditions officially called "syndromes" aren't the only ones vulnerable to such abuse. Many of the words we associate with "diseases" actually refer more to syndromes, because no one is sure whether they represent single entities. This really hit home one day when I attended a discussion of "genes and cancer" by several physicians at Harvard University's three hundred fiftieth birthday celebration. One of these doctors, Frederick Pei Li, a member since 1967 of the Clinical Epidemiology Branch of the National Cancer Institute and associate professor of medicine at the Dana-Farber Cancer Institute, emphasized that cancer is "not one disease but hundreds of diseases." What all these diseases share, added Dr. Philip Leder, the John Emory Andrus professor and chairman of the Department of Genetics at the Harvard Medical School, is "a disorder of growth." Cells with cancer do not appreciate the information available to limit their growth and development; their "control box" has been ripped out, and the affected cells are "on all the time."

And yet, Li went on to explain that each of these diseases called "cancer" is different, depending on the organ and type of cells involved. Thus, if the organ is the lung and the cells are the flat cells on the surface (squamous cells), then the disease may be "squamous-cell carcinoma of the lung." If the organ is the prostate and the type of cell is glandular, then the disease may be "adenocarcinoma of the prostate."

Both lung cancer and prostate cancer are forms of "cancer," of course; they share enough symptoms and signs (particularly uncontrolled cell growth) to give their condition a common name. Every day people talk about them—and hundreds of other cancers—in one breath, joining the "American Cancer Society," helping in the "fight against cancer," looking for a "cure for cancer." Nevertheless, lung cancer and prostate cancer, like most other forms of cancer, simply do not share enough traits to be lumped together as a single entity. As the average patient with lung cancer will attest, his cough, wheezing, and very short life expectancy are nothing at all like the bloody urine and bone pain of the average patient with prostate cancer, who may have his disease for years without noticing symptoms. The point is that a few shared characteristics may give patients a common name; that name, however, does not necessarily represent just one disease.

Epilepsy is another catchall term. As we saw earlier, patients with epilepsy have recurrent seizures, produced when certain neurons in the brain suddenly start firing ("discharging") excessively, but these "seizures" can occur in different ways: some people have seizures in different parts of the brain than others, while other people develop seizures because of distinct disorders of the brain or body. What is confusing, though, is that the different types of seizures occasionally overlap, suggesting that they may not be as different as we think.[15] Grand mal seizures, for example, can result when a partial seizure in a centralized group of neurons happens to spread to the entire brain. This phenomenon is considered a third form of epilepsy—"partial seizure with secondary generalization"—but the result can look identical to other forms; for whether the seizure started all over the brain or in some select group of cells, the patient is going to have a grand mal seizure.

Despite this similar appearance, not all grand mal seizures are necessarily the same disease. Because partial seizures seem to result from a structural abnormality (damaged neurons) they are called "symptomatic epilepsy"; that is, they are "symptoms" of a distinctly damaged part of the body. This category would include the grand mal seizures resulting from partial seizures with secondary generalization, since the problem can ultimately be traced to a specific structural abnormality. In contrast, a grand mal attack traceable to generalized seizures would be called "idiopathic epilepsy" because no one can explain why it happens; there is no obviously damaged group of neurons.

Obviously, this labeling implies very different groups of patients and treatment regimens: perhaps the people with symptomatic epilepsy, for example, can be helped in a more systematic way by aiming specific treatments at their damaged cells. Consequently, some doctors prefer to view "epilepsy" not as a single disease, but as a syndrome or symptom-complex made up of related but distinct conditions. The *Cecil Textbook of Medicine,* in fact, calls the chapter on this condition "The Epilepsies"—not "Epilepsy." [16] The author feels that the epilepsies are more like symptom-complexes (syndromes) than they are like one disease because, as with cancer, there are many different forms too dissimilar to warrant lumping all the patients together.

As commonly used, then, the names of many so-called diseases or conditions seem more like catchall terms for a variety of conditions and diseases. Calling someone "dyslexic" can mean he has anything from a mild reading problem to a severe handicap. Calling a child "hyperactive" or "hyperkinetic" can mean she has anything from a short attention span to brain damage. Still other "diseases," "disabilities," and "disorders" are defined more by what they are *not* than by what they *are.* Thus, learning disabilities are any "disorders in the understanding or processing of language, including difficulties in listening, thinking, talking, reading, or math" that are *not* primarily attributable to visual, aural, or motor handicaps, to mental retardation, to emotional disturbance, or to environmental disadvantages. [17] This sort of negative definition leaves a lot of room, then, for different kinds of conditions that can be called "learning disorders." The psychiatric profession has tried to circumvent such confusion among mental disorders by offering quite strict definitional criteria in their *Diagnostic and Statistical Manual of Mental Disorders;* but at the scientific meetings that I have attended as a medical journalist and in the research papers I have read, many of the investigations of specific mental disorders bypassed this source when defining patient populations, just as the patients themselves do when they hear certain labels applied to themselves.

One word of warning: just as the description of a medical condition need not include the term "syndrome" in order to be a syndrome, some conditions called "syndrome" may actually be diseases. In conditions such as Tourette syndrome (a neurological condition characterized by unpredictable tics, twitches, and involuntary, often scatological utterances) or Turner's syndrome (short stature, undeveloped gonads, and various other abnormalities associated with the absence of a second sex chromosome), the label "syndrome" is really just a vestigial term left over from days when less was known about the condition. For all intents and purposes, the medical profession considers these syndromes to be distinct diseases. The question in considering the status of any medical condition, then, is not whether it is called a syndrome (although this often helps), but whether or not it is legitimate to assume it is a single entity.

▲ LOVING SYNDROMES FOR THEMSELVES

As we have seen, lumping random symptoms together and calling them a "syndrome" serves some very useful functions in medicine. The hypothetical "chocolate ice cream syndrome" discussed at the beginning of the present chapter may be a catchall phrase that describes blonde women with big red spots on their left cheeks and uncontrollable hiccups who have just eaten chocolate ice cream but who can be cured with whipped cream. It's certainly easier to say "chocolate ice cream syndrome" than to detail each woman's specific symptoms. Moreover, some treatments work for all women with these symptoms, and certainly the relief of knowing that "it's not all in my head" justifies considering this condition as one "thing," at least until we know better. In short, without a little experimental lumping, all medicine would remain completely random and haphazard.

The problems outlined in the rest of the chapter, however, are the result of people jumping too soon from syndrome to disease. Some people do this because they forget that the option of syndrome is available to them. For example, the authors of a popular book on PMS propose that you either consider PMS a disease or you dismiss it as "all in the head." [18] They have no sympathy for the latter judgment, of course, since they show plenty of evidence that PMS has a real physical-psychological basis. But they neglect a third and quite reasonable possibility—that PMS is a catchall term for the many symptoms that can occur regularly in a woman's body in the days before her menstrual period. These symptoms may not have a common cause or common treatment, but they are all somehow related to the menstrual cycle.

This conclusion seems perfectly plausible. But drawing it actually requires an understanding that it is possible to feel bad without having a disease—at least according to the knowledge of the time. Perhaps PMS will one day turn out to be one disease; or, alternatively, it may turn out to be six diseases or a hundred diseases. Even though we don't know the ultimate conclusion, it is not necessary now to deny that many women experience symptoms premenstrually. The question is whether it's useful to lump all those symptoms together as one disease called "PMS," and, at present, that is a matter for debate.

In other words, just because something is not necessarily one disease doesn't mean that it's imaginary. It is justifiable to lump certain symptoms together and say that "present research does not allow us to determine whether these symptoms represent one disease or several— or a by-product of one or more other diseases—but this medical ignorance does not mitigate the discomfort that patients experience." There is nothing wrong about calling something a syndrome, but it is crucial to realize that this syndrome is not necessarily the same as a disease.

CHAPTER 7

How Diseases Come and Go

While turning symptoms and syndromes into diseases may be inappropriate, many symptoms, syndromes, and other unnamed conditions do become official diseases legitimately. By looking at what it takes for something to become a disease—and to stop being a disease, for that matter—the present chapter helps explain why there are so many nameless diseases and how some nameless diseases may eventually find names.

New diseases can appear for several reasons, the same reasons that can make other diseases disappear. Most simply, a new technique can reveal hitherto-unknown data that link unexplained phenomena. Here the disease always has existed to some extent but could not be recognized for technical reasons. In other cases, doctors lack modes of seeing rather than modes of technology: although the symptoms and conditions of the disease exist, doctors fail to recognize them; the disease comes into being when doctors stop viewing particular symptoms or events as irrelevant and start viewing them as part of a larger pattern. Finally, some diseases are truly new and never existed in the world or in a certain part of the world before—perhaps because a virus mutated or because a migrant population introduced a disease into a different region. Frequently, of course, more than one of these explanations accounts for the emergence or disappearance of a disease; but, generally, one reason predominates. With some of today's newest diseases, however, there hasn't been enough time to enable historical perspective to help untangle the intertwined explanations.[1]

▲ STAINS, MICROSCOPES, AND CURETTES

New diseases born out of new technical capabilities are the easiest to understand. In the seventeenth and eighteenth centuries, for example, new tools allowed doctors to "see" for the first time such diseases as chicken pox, whooping cough, scarlatina, ergotism, chlorosis, rickets, sciatica, and angina pectoris.[2] At first these discoveries arose rather haphazardly, but by the beginning of the eighteenth century the search for new diseases had become systematic. This search, in fact, was part of the various nosology schemes discussed above in Chapter 3 whereby physicians were trying to describe diseases as botanists described plants. Furthermore, as we saw, French doctors were defining new diseases by linking the lesions they found inside bodies with the symptoms they had seen in these same patients before death.[3] Thus, when Pierre-Fidèle Bretonneau (1778–1862) found that certain patients with sore throats also had thin, tough membranes covering their throats, he named a new disease: diphtheria.

Meanwhile, in the British Isles, a group of keen observers noted that certain anatomical and structural changes seemed to correspond to distinct laboratory findings; they, too, called these observations new diseases (and usually named them after themselves). Richard Bright (1789–1858), for example, combined three separate observations—shriveled kidneys, accumulation of fluid in the tissues ("dropsy"), and large amounts of albumin in the urine—to name the new disease "Bright's disease," which has come to mean a distinct form of chronic kidney inflammation.

Similarly, the discovery of pernicious anemia depended on improved tools for viewing and analyzing blood cells. This disease involves impaired red blood cell production owing to a deficiency of vitamin B_{12}. Today, pernicious anemia is easily treatable with regular injections of that vitamin; before the middle of the twentieth century, however, anyone with this disease had an often fatal condition whose agonizing symptoms included pallor, weakness, shortness of breath, sore mouth and tongue, tingling extremities, numbness, lack of balance, and dementia. According to David Steinberg, chief of the Section of Hematology at the Lahey Clinic in Burlington, Massachusetts, scientists didn't even know about red blood cells until the compound microscope was developed in the seventeenth century. Later, better stains, counting chambers, and colorimetric techniques allowed investigators to examine, count, and analyze blood cells well enough to distinguish several forms of anemia and to describe the large, oval-shaped red blood cells characteristic of pernicious anemia.[4] Only then did scientists have a definite entity and a reason to look for a treatment.

Combining distinct symptoms is not the only way to "discover" a new disease. Better tools also allow researchers to discriminate between conditions previously lumped together, often uncovering a new disease or two in the process. For example, when the Parisian doctor René-Théophile-Hyacinthe Laënnec (1781–1826) compared observations he made of his sick patients with observations of the lesions he discovered during their postmortem exams, he was able to divide the disease peripneumonia, known since ancient times, into numerous distinct diseases, including pneumonia, emphysema, and various forms of bronchitis.[5]

Technological changes have continued to create and abolish diseases in recent years. Consider endometriosis, for example. For centuries doctors had noticed that, for no apparent reason, certain women died during pregnancy—or never became pregnant at all, or suffered extreme pelvic pain.[6] According to the author Julia Older, "Your great-great-grandmother . . . might have been told the pain was because of her 'evil ways.'"

But then technology changed. In 1846 Joseph-Claude-Anthelme Recamier designed the curette for scraping the uterus—never before possible. In 1860 Karl Rokitansky described finding tissue that belonged inside the uterus on several internal organs, and a handful of researchers between 1860 and 1921 reported similar findings. Taken together, these studies suggested that in some women the tissue lining of the uterus that is normally expelled from the body during menstruation (i.e., the "endometrial tissue") goes awry: it travels outside the uterus and implants itself on the ovaries, the fallopian tubes, the outer walls of the uterus, the pelvic lining, the cervix, and/or the vagina.[7] These implants bleed monthly along with the uterus, often causing severe pain. In 1922, doctors gave this condition a name: endometriosis.[8] A new disease had come into being.

The creation of these "new" diseases—endometriosis, Bright's disease, and diphtheria—is easy enough to understand. Although people probably had suffered from these conditions for centuries, doctors simply hadn't had the tools to uncover them. Many are strictly physical processes with few behavioral components, and the key to their discovery was simply to develop and employ the right tools. Diphtheria couldn't have been defined without the ability to peer down throats and analyze lesions; Bright's disease couldn't have been recognized without laboratory techniques that detected albumin in the urine; and endometriosis couldn't have been recognized as a physical problem until someone developed the curette. Undoubtedly there are many unexplained symptoms and conditions floating around today which are misidentified as "all in the head" or "nonexistent" simply because we lack the tools to identify them as diseases.

Conversely, there are undoubtedly people walking around with diseases that will one day disappear, and not from better treatment. Improved technology can eliminate as well as create diseases. Until the end of the nineteenth century, medical texts often referred to a disease known as "the whites" or "fluor albus." Today we would regard the described conditions as a conglomeration of various diseases and symptoms, but for some eighteenth- and nineteenth-century practitioners, "the whites" represented a unified problem. The disease, distinguished from venereal disease, involved a white vaginal discharge and often appeared at distinct times of the month. When Dr. John Gunn described this disease in his popular treatise, read widely by laypeople for decades following its original 1830 publication, he attributed it to various causes, including impaired

> powers of the womb . . . severe labours, repeated miscarriages, getting out of bed too soon after child-birth; or by taking cold at this time, or any other time when the menses or courses are about coming on; or by over fatigue or weakness, produced by general bad health; or where the general secretions and excretions have been deranged by disease.

Because Gunn is not known as an original medical thinker, we may presume that his view of "the whites" was a fairly common one among practitioners and patients of his day. Gunn divided "the whites" into stages. In the first stage, the vaginal discharges resemble egg white and have no smell and little color. This description sounds very much like what today is regarded as either normal vaginal discharges at certain times of the month—especially since Gunn observes their periodic appearance—or as leukorrhea (a whitish vaginal discharge), which is not a disease in itself but a symptom of various diseases and which, toward the end of the century, became the preferred term for "the whites." True, Gunn's first stage may have been accompanied by backache, irregular menstruation, and shooting pains—but all of these we today might dismiss as common symptoms very likely unrelated to normal discharges or leukorrhea (indeed, the term "fluor albus" is today synonymous with leukorrhea). In 1830, however, these women would have to regard their normal cervical changes as a sign of this ghastly disease, one with the potential to enter a secondary stage in which discharges become yellow and offensive-smelling and then a third stage in which discharges become greenish, tough, gluey, and even more malodorous. Again, these latter cases might be categorized as part of many different and unrelated diseases today—including nonspecific vaginal infections, trichomoniasis vaginalis (a parasitical infection), and even gonorrhea, each with different treatments and worries. In the worst stage of "the whites"—which Gunn says will occur if the disease is neglected—the discharges are very "offensive," mixed with blood, and

> the face becomes of a sickly greenish hue; under the eye there is an unnatural color; the lips become purple; the feet and legs swell; the face becomes subject to flushes of heat; there is a dry cough and great difficulty of breathing, particularly on the slightest exertion; and unless relief is obtained, the disease will, *after this stage,* terminate either in CONSUMPTION or DROPSY.

To avoid this dreadful fate, then, women who may have had a condition—that is, a normal vaginal discharge—that we wouldn't consider a disease at all today were advised to cleanse their "private parts" with cold water many times a day and to douche with cold water and "lead water," to sleep on a hard bed, to rise early, and to take mild laxatives and various other drugs (including turpentine). As the condition worsened, so did the remedies.[9]

"The whites" eventually disappeared as a disease when improved microscopic capabilities allowed doctors to see that discharges which otherwise looked identical could actually represent many different conditions. Here, then, technological change eliminated a disease by splitting it up. Technological change can also eliminate a disease by merging it with a different disease. Consider puerperal fever ("childbed fever"), for example, an often fatal condition, feared since ancient Greece, that afflicted women after childbirth. By the mid-nineteenth century, up to 10 percent of women who delivered in certain hospitals and clinics were dying of this "disease." Explanations varied, although they generally turned on the woman's bad health habits or on pure chance. Nevertheless, by the second half of the nineteenth century, some doctors were suggesting that puerperal fever was spread by germs on the hands of the doctors themselves. They pointed out that doctors would handle corpses or treat patients with various infections and then, without washing their hands, proceed to deliver babies. Although most of the medical community refused to believe these accusations, by the 1870s investigators were able to demonstrate that certain bacteria, including those causing the diseases erysipelas and scarlet fever, were responsible for the infections following childbirth.[10] Thus, what had been thought of as a separate disease for thousands of years turned out to be another form of an already recognized bacterial infection.

▲ NEW WAYS OF SEEING

Other new diseases arise—or disappear—because their existence depends as much on the way current society views the problem as it does on new discoveries. These diseases, which often have behavioral symptoms, are molded by the way different groups of people see the same phenomena: while some will see a condition and call it a moral affliction, sin, or even normal behavior, others will call it a disease. In other words, defining a new disease has to do with changes in values or worldview. New technology often plays a role, but the underlying reason why doctors discover a new disease is that the condition fits current explanations of what constitutes a disease. In other words, these new diseases are born not when some new medical fact arises, but when some official agency or even a private company (such as a pharmaceutical company) decides that the correct way of seeing is to call the problem a disease.

Today's society, for example, is much more willing than some previous societies to look for physical or genetic explanations of moods and behaviors and, if possible, to call them diseases rather than sins. Thus, some of today's new diseases were recognized long ago but were seen as conditions that reflected sin and moral degradation. A changed attitude, combined with some biological explanation uncovered by new technology, allows the medical profession to appropriate the condition and to name the old "feeling" or "behavior" a true "disease."

Early-nineteenth-century doctors, however, thought almost in reverse: instead of attributing behaviors and emotions to physical abnormalities, they often attributed physical abnormalities to behaviors or emotions—or to morality. For example, alcoholism, like many other physical problems, had "moral" or "psychological" roots. According to Dr. Gunn, whose views, again, reflected the common beliefs of his day, people developed alcoholism if they had a disorder of the passion known as "intemperance," and the result was a disease of the mind, parallel to but not equivalent to a physical disease. Gunn argued that you could remove the drunkard's bottle or administer helpful drugs, but there was no way these physical measures could get to the basic problem. As Gunn put it in 1830, you cannot fundamentally help the patient unless you "adapt your means to the original nature of the disease; you must employ the *moral powers* of dissuasive eloquence; the divine *consolations* of RELIGION."[11]

As the years went by, arguments like this became more deeply ingrained, and people thought of alcoholism as a moral affliction, not a disease at all. Indeed, only recently has the psychiatric profession decided differently. Studies suggest that dependence on alcohol isn't a matter of discipline at all: certain people simply cannot drink alcohol without becoming dependent on it and allowing it to seriously disrupt their lives. Of course, the exact reason for this dependence remains unknown, but modern researchers know that many behaviors have physical explanations; thus, they can attribute them to genes or biochemistry rather than to morals—an approach that didn't fit early-nineteenth-century views of behavior.[12] And so, although people with alcoholism in the late twentieth century have had problems identical to those of people with alcoholism in 1830, only the former have had a disease—all because authorities decided to classify it that way. Nothing else has changed.

Our society's taste for biochemical explanations, rather than moral ones, can also be seen in a new disease (or potentially new disease) that primarily involves emotions. Since ancient times, some people have noted that they feel particularly depressed during the gray, winter months. Formerly, such feelings were of no medical concern: perhaps these people felt unhappy because they were thinking about how they couldn't swim in the lake, or how they would have to be shut up in a little room with their screaming children for months on end, or how much they missed the sun's warm rays. In any case, it was thought, clearly this mood wasn't a disease; it was just a case of letting your bad thoughts get the better of you. You had a moral problem or poor self-control.

In the past few years, however, a group of psychiatrists has offered a different explanation. Like several leading psychiatrists before them, they observed that during the winter months some patients have a very distinct group of symptoms: they tend to sleep more, have less energy, gain weight, and crave carbohydrates. For some psychiatrists today, these behaviors constitute a distinct condition, which they call "seasonal affective disorder," or SAD. People with hypothyroidism have similar symptoms—but year round; in contrast, the SAD patients are extremely happy and energetic during the summer. Similarly, patients described as having classic manic depression also share these symptoms, but their mood swings are generally random—not seasonal.

Those psychiatrists who believe that SAD is a distinct disease point out that there are many seasonal variations in animal behavior, such as hibernation, reproduction, and migration. In fact, animal studies have shown that all these behaviors are controlled by aspects of the environment, especially light and temperature, that produce chemical and hormonal changes and ultimately affect behavior. Something similar might be happening to SAD patients, these psychiatrists contend. The environment common in summer might be triggering one emotional state, while the winter environment might trigger another, perhaps through the variation in daylight hours. This isn't so farfetched—rats, for example, are more active at night, particularly around dawn and dusk, and when the nights grow longer, the rats have more hours of activity.

Other clues relating this condition directly to the season and sun level come from some preliminary studies showing that SAD patients can be helped with phototherapy: expose them to high levels of light, and they start feeling good. Furthermore, patients with SAD living closer to the equator report milder symptoms than those living farther away from it—north or south.[13] Finally, studies are beginning to suggest that levels of the hormone melatonin might decrease abnormally in SAD patients when light levels are particularly low, ultimately affecting their mood.

It's only these kinds of findings that have made it possible for psychiatrists to consider classifying SAD as a distinct psychiatric disorder. Two hundred years ago, there was no way to measure levels of melatonin, and no one had done studies to suggest that animals—or humans—could be controlled by light levels. That way of thinking just wasn't part of science, so no one "discovered" SAD. But if today's psychiatrists have their way, SAD will become a subtype of mood disorder, defined not by the exact symptoms but by the *pattern* of symptoms: namely, at least two consecutive years of depression that begins in the fall and ends in the spring. In this way, SAD resembles PMS and puerperal mental illness, both of which share symptoms with other diseases but which may be distinct because of unique timing. One of the reasons why all of these conditions are having trouble establishing their disease footing is that most psychiatrists—and doctors in general—are not in the habit of using the timing of symptoms, rather than the symptoms themselves, to define disease. As doctors start thinking more in this way, entities such as SAD, PMS, and puerperal mental illness are likely to be more easily accepted as distinct diseases.

Sometimes the decision to "make" a condition an official disease or disorder occurs—or doesn't occur—for purely political reasons. According to the psychiatrist Arthur Kleinman, for example, during the Cultural Revolution in China, Mao Zedong decided that mental illnesses such as depression were not so much diseases as wrong political thinking.[14] Similarly, while in the process of revising their official diagnostic manual, the American Psychiatric Association decided to compromise with feminist groups by relegating PMS (as well as two types of disturbed personalities) to the appendix of that manual. The feminist groups didn't want PMS listed at all, contending that calling PMS a psychiatric disorder would stigmatize women whose problems were biological (thus ignoring the fact that many psychiatric disorders happen to have biological origins). Putting PMS in the appendix was not entirely satisfactory, but feminist concerns definitely served to diminish the status of PMS as a psychiatric "disease" compared to conditions such as schizophrenia or depression.[15]

On the other hand, other new diseases arise when a distinctive attitude leads researchers to start "seeing" something that's not actually there—another reason (and a good one) why proposals of new diseases are often met with suspicion. A certain way of thinking about the meaning of disease actually leads to the discovery of what doctors who think differently cannot see at all. In the second half of the nineteenth century, for example, the disease "hysteria," which had been known in various forms to physicians, priests, and witch-hunters since Hippocrates, acquired a brand-new meaning.[16] Today we consider hysteria ("conversion disorder") to be a form of neurosis that may have symptoms including emotional instability, pain and tenderness around the ovaries, spine, and head, convulsions, retention of urine, fever, paralysis, choking sensations, and dimmed vision. Although some of these symptoms are "physical," today's doctors consider hysteria to be not a neurological disease, but an emotional disorder characterized largely by anxiety.

But in the mid-nineteenth century, doctors had different ideas. They saw a number of women showing hysterical symptoms, and suddenly it made sense to classify all these behaviors as part of a full-fledged neurological disease. The conventional wisdom was changing, and these doctors believed that behaviors and emotions had physical roots, rather than vice versa. Such an idea made a lot of sense at the time: after all, many French researchers were linking external symptoms with internal lesions, so why shouldn't mental conditions have similar links? These doctors therefore suspected that "hysteria" had some anatomical explanation; that is, they believed there was some underlying lesion or defect in brain tissue that accounted for the strange behavior. Indeed, for most of its history, doctors assumed that hysterical behavior stemmed from some sort of diseased internal part—first a "wandering" or "poisoned" womb, and later a "weak" head or nervous system. What's important to remember, though, is that even in the mid-nineteenth century the idea about hysteria's anatomical basis wasn't drawn from experimental data; it just happened to fit current neurological doctrine.

Not surprisingly, then, the neurologists of the time set out to verify this idea. And whether consciously or not, a number of investigators had such strong presuppositions that they did indeed find what they called the "hysterical lesion"—even documenting their findings with photographs. All of this documentation has not held up to the test of time, however, for no one today can find any brain lesion corresponding to hysterical behavior. Although today's doctors are also fond of looking for links between behavior and physical lesions, no one so far has authenticated the earlier findings about hysteria. Yet, the belief that hysteria was a disease with an anatomical basis was so strong in the mid-1800s that even the famed neurologist Jean-Martin Charcot (1825–1893) used these findings to describe the exact nature of the disease "hysteria," from its early stages to its final delirium.[17]

The new "attitude" that leads people to see a new "disease" can be economic as well as political or theoretical. Most commonly, a new drug or surgical technique will emerge, and an enterprising physician or pharmaceutical company will find some new medical problem which, like so many problems in other areas of life, arises only when a solution to it is available. Consider the account of the recent birth of the disease "shortness," as recounted by an article in the *New York Times Magazine*. According to this article, only after the biotechnology company Genentech had developed a way to synthesize abundant quantities of HGH (human growth hormone) did certain doctors, biotechnologists, parents, and businesspeople begin to regard "shortness" as a disease. Naturally occurring HGH is a hormone produced by the pituitary gland, responsible for stimulating bone growth. Administered to children with HGH deficiencies, the synthetic version of this hormone has been shown to add as many as eighteen inches to predicted adult heights. But according to the article's author, Barry Werth, Genentech went on to pursue children who were short (in the lowest three percentiles for height) but not deficient in growth hormone; often, the "patients" were otherwise unremarkable children who simply happened to have short parents. Werth quotes Dr. John D. Lanto of the Center for Clinical Medical Ethics at the University of Chicago's Pritzker School of Medicine as saying: "Until growth hormone came along, no one called normal shortness a disease. . . . It's become a disease only because a manipulation has become available, and because doctors and insurance companies, in order to rationalize their actions, have had to perceive it as one." With the recent finding that HGH may also slow signs of aging in elderly men, the economic interests of some pharmaceutical companies may soon lead to the view that "aging" is a disease as well.[18]

▲ DISEASES THAT REAPPEAR

Of course, sometimes the research inspired by a new way of thinking also turns out to be verified by later generations; the result is a new disease that emerges because of both a change in perspective and a change in medical knowledge. And, like hysteria, these changes over the years can make a disease come and go—or come, go, and come back again.

New diseases like puerperal mental illness and Tourette syndrome, for example, existed for a while, disappeared, and then returned.[19] As we have already seen, doctors in the first half of the nineteenth century recognized puerperal mental illness as a distinct disease. For the past hundred years or so, however, psychiatry texts and training programs have largely ignored these same symptoms and have refused to separate them from nonpuerperal conditions or to recognize them as distinct disorders.[20] In fact, even today the American Psychiatric Association's *Diagnostic and Statistical Manual of Mental Disorders* (DSM-III) describes puerperal psychosis as only an "atypical psychosis" and states that it does "not meet the criteria for an organic mental disorder, schizophreniaform disorder, paranoid disorder, or affective disorder." And yet, if groups like the Marcé Society, established in 1980 to help further research in this area, have their way, psychiatrists will once again recognize puerperal psychosis as a distinct mental illness.

Similarly, Tourette syndrome was fully recognized as a distinct condition as far back as 1885, the year that Charcot's pupil Georges Gilles de la Tourette (1857–1904) described it.[21] Patients with Tourette syndrome had excessive "nervous energy," which led them to make all sorts of undesirable movements ranging from tics, jerks, and grimaces to shrieks and curses. And yet, Tourette syndrome essentially "disappeared" in the first half of this century, when doctors scarcely reported it at all. Some physicians, indeed, regarded the condition as a product of Tourette's imagination; most had never heard of it. Only in the past decade or so have studies of neurotransmitters, publicized by groups such as the Tourette Syndrome Association, helped doctors to see, once again, that Tourette syndrome is a very real neurological condition.

How can we explain these shifting points of view? Like hysteria, the fate of both puerperal mental illness and Tourette syndrome can be understood by looking at the underlying medical beliefs of the day: if the diseases fit the predetermined notions, they were recognized; when they ceased to fit, they suddenly ceased to exist.

Renowned psychiatrists of the 1840s and 1850s not only believed in puerperal mental illness, but they could give detailed accounts of the symptoms and even enumerate subtypes.[22] In those years, it made sense to link emotional and physical complaints, even though doctors then may have preferred to say that the emotions were primary. It also made sense to consider the specific conditions (e.g., childbirth) surrounding a patient's complaints. But, even then, a few doctors were wondering: "Why have something called puerperal mental illness when it looks just like other kinds of mental illness? Just because it happens right after childbirth doesn't necessarily make it a distinct disease. After all, when measles happens right after childbirth, we don't call it puerperal measles."[23]

As the years went by, this point of view became more credible. Psychiatrists were becoming unhappy with the way they thought about diseases; doctors in other branches of medicine were finding very specific etiological agents—such as bacteria—at the heart of their diseases, and psychiatrists wanted an equally precise system. Emil Kraepelin therefore suggested a classification scheme that would define each psychiatric disease according to its etiology or at least according to some specifically damaged tissue: there had to be an easily detectable biological basis, not just a list of behaviors (hence the search for a hysterical lesion). In other words, psychiatrists hoped to explain and classify mental problems by means of physical phenomena—rather than vice versa. The trouble was, this kind of change couldn't work at the time. Knowledge of mental illness was just too limited, so psychiatrists often moved to the next best thing: they defined diseases as broad constellations of symptoms that often occurred together ("syndromes"), with no natural boundaries between them.[24]

But mental illness after childbirth did not fit nicely into this scheme either; it did not really constitute a syndrome. After all, the "constellation of symptoms" looked very much like the one seen in patients with manic depression or schizophrenia; the only difference had to do with the timing. Clearly, though, the current psychiatric classification scheme took no account of timing or circumstances: all that mattered were the symptoms. Thus, the easiest solution, notes the psychiatrist James A. Hamilton, was simply to expunge puerperal mental illness from the list of distinct diseases and to consider it as representing psychiatric conditions having the same symptoms. That's all there was to it; there was no longer any condition known as puerperal mental illness.

Other developments in society compounded neglect, according to Hamilton. First of all, as late-nineteenth-century physicians began to specialize, puerperal mental illness, being a hybrid condition composed of psychiatric as well as obstetrical components, started to slip between the cracks.[25] With the symptoms lying midway between obstetrics and psychiatry, psychiatrists and obstetricians alike tended to neglect postpartum mental problems. Furthermore, the severe cases that occurred were so evenly dispersed throughout the population that no one psychiatrist saw more than a few of them—so, if psychiatrists hadn't learned about this condition in medical school, they weren't likely to notice anything unusual. Besides, because patients suffering from postpartum mental illness usually shared symptoms with victims of several more standard varieties of mental illness, most psychiatrists until recently were likely to regard them "as if they were run-of-the-mill schizophrenics or manic-depressives."[26]

Only now, as psychiatry at last moves toward classifying diseases according to their biological basis rather than their symptoms, is puerperal psychosis creeping back into the picture. Some psychiatrists now estimate that about one in every thousand formerly normal women develop severely debilitating mental illness after childbirth and require psychiatric hospital care. In addition, perhaps one-tenth of all childbearing women suffer from postpartum depression—which may or may not be a separate condition. Sometimes mothers will harbor indifferent, hostile, or even murderous feelings toward their infants. Finally, 50 to 70 percent of women probably experience "maternity blues" or "transient mild depression" in the first few days after delivery.[27]

Premenstrual syndrome's Dr. Katharina Dalton hypothesizes that these mood swings may be related to hormonal changes. During the menstrual cycle, she says, moods are affected by hormonal changes that, compared to the ones following childbirth, are infinitesimal. During pregnancy, hormones like progesterone increase massively, and the abrupt deprivation of these hormones after delivery may result in a sort of "drug withdrawal" behavior. In fact, Dalton adds, although administering progesterone won't relieve other forms of depression, it may help postpartum depression.[28]

Interestingly, now that psychiatrists like James Hamilton, who has been actively campaigning for the recognition of puerperal mental illness for several decades, recognize the biological basis of that disease, they are also able to point out unique symptoms which differentiate it from other mental illnesses. In other words, contrary to the classifiers of a hundred years ago, puerperal mental illness does *not* look exactly like textbook manic-depressive psychosis or schizophrenia. First of all, argues Hamilton, puerperal patients change moods and relapse more frequently than other patients. They also tend to have concurrent physical complaints, such as weakness, pallor, anemia, stomach upset, sweating, menstrual irregularity, circulation problems, and abnormal uterine cells—problems not usually seen in other mental patients. And, finally, people with classic schizophrenia rarely show such symptoms as delirium, confusion, hallucination, and drastic mood swings, all common in postpartum women who otherwise seem to have schizophrenia or some other severe disorder of mood and behavior.

The story of Tourette syndrome is amazingly similar. For late-nineteenth-century neurologists, this syndrome made perfect sense, just as puerperal psychosis had to their predecessors. As we have already seen with hysteria, contemporary theories often united physical problems such as nerve damage with unusual moods or behaviors. The neurologist Oliver Sacks writes that, for Georges Gilles de la Tourette and his peers, "this syndrome was a sort of possession by primitive impulses and urges . . . a possession with an organic base—a very definite (if undiscovered) neurological disorder." According to Sacks, the syndrome represented a struggle between a "soul" that wanted one thing and a "body" that wanted another; in a sense, these primitive impulses were constantly battling with the normal brain. As with puerperal mental illness in the mid-nineteenth century, many doctors published papers on this syndrome, and others were able to distinguish different forms of the condition.

Over the years, however, the field of neurology changed, and Tourette's old theory was no longer an acceptable way to define a disease. Neurologists and psychiatrists stopped believing that diseases could be made up of "soul" and "body" components: if the problem was in the "soul" (mind), then it belonged to the field of psychiatry; if the problem was in the "body" (brain), it belonged to neurology. Tourette syndrome, having aspects of both body and soul, belonged nowhere, just as puerperal mental illness had belonged neither to psychiatry nor to obstetrics. And so, Tourette syndrome "disappeared" (even though people certainly suffered from it).

But again, in the past decade or so, medical thinking has undergone yet another shift. Neurologists increasingly are coming to understand that many seemingly behavioral problems, problems of the mind or soul, actually have their origin in a disturbed neurotransmitter (a chemical that transmits signals between brain cells). In other words, once again mind and body have been linked. Thus, findings are beginning to suggest that Tourette syndrome might be a real disease, related somehow to chemical imbalance in the regions of the brain that control basic emotions and instincts. In 1974, some fifty crusaders founded the Tourette Syndrome Association (TSA), and by the early 1980s the ranks had grown to several thousand.[29]

Through the urgings of the TSA, much like the urgings of puerperal mental illness's Marcé Society, Tourette syndrome has once again become a legitimate medical condition. Not that the fight for recognition doesn't continue: many doctors, trained by the textbooks of long ago, still don't know about it. People still complain about going from doctor to doctor and having their symptoms attributed to "nervousness," "mental illness," "allergies," and "family problems" until they read some literature from the TSA (or popular advice columns like Ann Landers') and seek out a doctor who is up-to-date in the field of neurology. Until medical education improves and someone writes these new diseases into all the textbooks, then, puerperal mental illness and Tourette syndrome will, in a sense, still not be full-fledged "diseases."

▲ OUT-OF-THE-BLUE DISEASES

Finally, there are a few truly new diseases, new because they never existed before and not because they couldn't have been discovered or because they didn't conform to contemporary medical thinking. One medical historian, Robert P. Hudson, identifies three types of such new diseases, which ultimately result from human activity:

1 *Environmental diseases.* These "are born when human beings engage in certain activities . . . [and] die when those activities cease or when people take whatever precautions are necessary to separate their physiology from the offending agents."
2 *Iatrogenic diseases.* These conditions, resulting from medical practice, have mechanisms basically identical to those underlying the environmental diseases. They "are born when patients encounter new diagnostic or therapeutic modalities . . . [and] die when the contact ends."
3 *Cultural diseases.* These are associated with lifestyle and include such diseases as cirrhosis from alcohol, lung cancer and emphysema from cigarettes, trichinosis from undercooked pork and beef, kuru from cannibalism, and hookworm from going barefoot.[30]

These sorts of diseases depend on specific man-made conditions and can change; they therefore exist only when conditions are ripe. Other types of out-of-the-blue diseases, however, are more stubborn and seem to live on forever once born.

At around the turn of the century, a new disease called "Savill's disease" arose out of the blue and, interestingly enough, lasted only a short number of years. Indeed, this disease existed only in certain infirmaries of late-nineteenth-century London. Thomas Dixon Savill (1856–1910), medical superintendent of the Poor Law infirmary in the London borough of Paddington from 1885 to 1892, noticed in the summer of 1891 that many elderly paupers developed what seemed to be a new, sometimes fatal epidemic skin disease, characterized by inflamed, peeling, flaking, brownish skin. Poor Law infirmaries housed the sickest, oldest, and most destitute citizens, many of whom came down with the new disease. In milder cases only the face, arms, and hands were afflicted, but the whole body would suffer in the more severe cases. Furthermore, Dr. Savill reported that patients gave off an offensive odor and had inflamed, painful eyes and throats. A little over a tenth of them died from the disease. Still, there was rarely any fever, and in six to eight weeks most patients recovered.

This pattern seemed to represent an entirely new condition. The peeling skin suggested eczema and other common skin complaints, but none of these diseases was infectious like the new disease. The new disease also looked a bit like pityriasis rubra and scarlatina but lacked most other symptoms of those complaints. Stranger still, the disease recurred in a very limited area—in at least five London infirmaries during the summer or early autumn of each year until 1894. The historian M. A. Crowther estimates that there were at least 467 cases reported during 1891–1893, and probably 240 more in 1894. A Scottish poorhouse reported a similar disease in 1888/89, but otherwise all cases of Savill's disease occurred in London, nearly all in the infirmaries for paupers.

Only after years of investigation did Savill's successors come up with an explanation: Savill's disease resulted from adulterated milk served to susceptible patients living in particularly unhygienic conditions; once laws had been passed to ensure better inspection of dairies and infirmaries, Savill's disease ceased to exist. The milk may have been infected with bacteria or may have even contained poison. Crowther notes that the most severe form of the disease attacked only very susceptible groups—the elderly and the infirm—"and since Poor Law infirmaries were the most common receptacles for these groups, the disease was noticed only there." No new cases were reported after 1903, by which time the quality of milk was under public control and refrigeration was used much more frequently.[31]

It's hard to know now whether Dr. Savill saw a truly unique phenomenon—there are no patients left to test—but the historical evidence suggests that he may well have. What is clear, in any case, is that this new and short-lived disease could only have existed when certain other conditions were ripe: Poor Law infirmaries (which contained large numbers of sick, old, and unhygienic residents), unregulated milk supplies, and inadequate refrigeration. Before the Poor Law infirmaries existed, there was no Savill's disease; and after milk supplies were better controlled, there was no Savill's disease. But for a few years, a truly unique disease seems to have existed.

Other new diseases may arise when a virus mutates to some new form. This may be what happened in the case of AIDS, which, notwithstanding its label as a "syndrome," is not only a new disease but a new *kind* of disease: it is a thing in itself (a disease associated with a specific virus and a specific phenomenon—immunosuppression), but some of its symptoms are actually diseases as well. In other words, AIDS is a disease made up of several other diseases.

To understand this situation, let's look back at how AIDS came to be a disease. Back in 1979 no one had heard of AIDS. But a few doctors started noticing some very unusual events, which led to them to publish several mysterious reports in 1981. In June of that year, to begin with, doctors at the UCLA School of Medicine and the Cedars Mt. Sinai Hospital in Los Angeles reported that five young homosexual men had developed *Pneumocystis carinii* pneumonia (PCP). This disease itself isn't so rare, but seeing it in young, previously healthy men was truly bizarre. An "opportunistic infection," PCP normally takes the "opportunity" only to infect people whose immune systems already function poorly. Even stranger, these five patients, two of whom died during treatment, had other opportunistic infections that were normally seen only in organ-transplant patients whose immune systems have been broken down intentionally (to prevent rejection of the new organ). This report alarmed doctors: healthy young men were not supposed to develop opportunistic infections.

Alarm increased when, a month later, Dr. Alvin Friedman and colleagues described the twenty-six young homosexual men they had seen as patients since early 1979 in New York and California. These men all had Kaposi's sarcoma, which, at the time, was a rare malignancy in this country.[32] Interestingly, several of these patients also had PCP, just like the five California men described above. More disturbingly, within two years of the diagnosis of Kaposi's sarcoma, eight of the twenty-six young men had died.

Nor did the mystery end there. A few months later, another eleven inexplicable cases of PCP were reported in California among young homosexual men or drug abusers, none of whom would have been suspected to develop this disease. And two of these men had Kaposi's sarcoma as well![33]

How to explain these coincidences? Doctors almost immediately suspected some link between the PCP and the Kaposi's sarcoma cases, partly because several men had developed both diseases. Furthermore, with no common environmental toxin identified, doctors tried to find something that all these men shared. A few religious zealots shouted, "Homosexuality, of course, that's the root of their problems. God is punishing them all." Researchers, however, proposed a more plausible explanation: all these men were susceptible to opportunistic infections, developing many different kinds of fungal, viral, and mycobacterial infections that normally don't afflict healthy young people. Perhaps, then, they were all suffering from some unknown *process* that interfered with the ability to fight off infection. Some doctors even narrowed the explanation to some sort of cytomegalovirus, perhaps spread through sexual contact, since these organisms had been known to depress the immune system. On the other hand, if the immune systems of these men were depressed for some other reason, they might have been susceptible to picking up the cytomegalovirus afterward. Thus, no one could be sure which came first—the virus or the depressed immune system.[34]

All that doctors could say in 1981, then, was that there might have been a common link between the occurrence of these *diverse diseases* and that this link somehow involved a poorly working immune system. But there was no evidence yet that this link represented the one disease we now know as AIDS; instead, all that existed were a few diseases such as Kaposi's sarcoma and PCP which were occurring when they shouldn't have been occurring.

Over the next few years, however, these strange but separate diseases, together with the shared immunodeficiency, fused together to form a new syndrome: acquired immunodeficiency syndrome, or AIDS.[35] By calling AIDS a syndrome (some called it a disease, too, or both a syndrome and a disease), researchers were forging an explanation for the mysteries of 1981. They had hypothesized a single process which alone accounted for the unusual occurrences of many different infections. By August 1983 more than 2,000 cases of this new syndrome had been reported in the United States, together with 122 cases from at least twenty other countries.[36] Most of the cases occurred among four major risk groups: homosexual or bisexual men; intravenous drug abusers; Haitians living in the United States; and people with hemophilia. Researchers hypothesized that AIDS had originated in equatorial Africa and had somehow transmigrated to Haiti. It then appeared in New York City and, the following year, in San Francisco. By 1984, doctors estimated that the number of new cases in the United States began to rise at a rate that doubled every six months.

By compiling statistics about what happened to people with "AIDS" and by talking about the people who developed "AIDS," furthermore, the American medical profession (and public) had begun to think of this phenomenon as one entity, a single process—in short, as a unique disease. In 1984, Anthony S. Fauci, chief of the Laboratory of Immunoregulation at the National Institute of Allergy and Infectious Diseases, wrote that AIDS is a "new disease" whose cause is unknown but which is almost surely attributable to a transmissible agent, most likely a virus. He noted that mortality may well approach 100 percent, "making this one of the most extraordinary transmissible *diseases* in history" (emphasis added).[37]

Forces quickly gathered to fight this unusual new "disease." In late 1985, Secretary of Health and Human Services Margaret M. Heckler noted that within the past few years every agency within the U.S. Public Health Service—the Alcohol, Drug Abuse, and Mental Health Administration; the Centers for Disease Control; the Food and Drug Administration; the Health Resources and Services Administration; and the National Institutes of Health—had joined the front lines. By late 1985, $189.9 million in federal monies had been committed to support governmental, academic, and private research efforts. "Never in the history of medicine," wrote Heckler, "has so much been learned about an entirely new *disease* in such a short time" (emphasis added).[38]

But AIDS was an extraordinary disease in yet another way: it consisted of subsets of conditions (Kaposi's sarcoma and PCP, for example) that formerly existed as diseases in their own right. And yet, with the new evidence coming out of New York and California, doctors no longer found it useful to think of a patient as suffering from PCP— even though that patient may indeed have been infected with the *Pneumocystis carinii* organism and have all the symptoms of PCP. It was now simply more useful to say that this patient had AIDS. It told doctors more about him: namely, that he not only had this one infection but that he was susceptible to other infections and might very well die in the next few years. On the other hand, if an old man who had just had a transplant operation developed PCP, doctors would probably say he just had PCP; there would have been no reason to suspect AIDS. But again, in the case of a young man infected with *P. carinii,* the very same symptoms suddenly belonged to an entirely new disease or, rather, to two diseases at once. The same can be said of people who had any of the other opportunistic infections characteristic of AIDS: they really had two diseases simultaneously, but it was more useful in terms of treatment and prognosis to think of them as having AIDS.

All this may have seemed like a strange way to think about diseases, but it did explain a lot about the mysterious occurrences of the past few years. It didn't explain everything, though; after all, there were many different ways to "have AIDS." One person could have Kaposi's sarcoma and have AIDS, while another could have PCP and have AIDS; the only thing they'd have in common was a compromised immune system and an opportunistic infection—but not necessarily the same opportunistic infection. Some AIDS patients had severe symptoms and died almost immediately; others lingered on for years. No definitive test could confirm AIDS; each test only confirmed some other specific disease which, together with other clues (such as young age, membership in a risk group, or no evidence of previous immunological compromise), suggested AIDS.[39] Was AIDS really one disease, then? doctors asked. Could so many different manifestations really stem from one underlying defect?[40]

The answer came when researchers discovered a virus that was shared by all AIDS victims. Suddenly this strange disease made up of other diseases and having no concrete definition began to take shape. At last, the "guess" that AIDS really was a unique disease started making much more sense. In 1984, independent researchers at the Institut Pasteur in Paris and at the National Cancer Institute in Bethesda, Maryland, revealed a specific infectious "cause" of AIDS, a retrovirus now called HIV (the human immunodeficiency virus). At last, AIDS had a characteristic that differentiated it from any of the diseases it comprised. Patients with AIDS not only had certain signs and symptoms, but they all had been exposed to one and only one virus, probably a virus that never existed before.

Legionnaire's disease represents another example of a new disease that probably arose because a new infective agent had appeared on the scene. The first cases appeared in the 1960s or earlier, but nobody noticed them until years later because they basically resembled other forms of pneumonia.[41] But in 1976, when more than two hundred delegates at an American Legion convention in Philadelphia came down with pneumonia all at once and twenty-nine died, eyebrows couldn't help rising. Pneumonia, after all, does not normally occur in epidemic outbreaks. It usually occurs sporadically in people who are already ill with viral infections or who have other predisposing conditions such as alcoholism, malnutrition, or general weakness. And yet, the lung infection, chest pain, dry cough, high fever, and chills all made this disease look very much like common bacterial pneumonia.

Investigators at the Centers for Disease Control in Atlanta got cracking and eventually found an explanation. This "pneumonia" was no ordinary pneumonia; rather, the new condition—"Legionnaire's disease"—seemed to be linked to an unknown bacterium that had been isolated from the lung of a Legionnaire. Investigators later found high levels of antibodies to this bacterium in the blood of the survivors—and in the blood of those who had survived several strange forms of pneumonia during previous years. The bacterium, named *Legionella pneumophila,* is very difficult to stain and identify, which might help explain the trouble researchers had in recognizing it as a cause of pneumonia. In fact, some small studies are now suggesting that one in six adults admitted to the hospital with "pneumonia" really has Legionnaire's disease.[42] Of course, before anyone knew to look for *L. pneumophila*—and before it even existed!—no one could have known that these patients didn't have one of the same kinds of pneumonia that had been around for years.

Further investigation showed that Legionnaire's disease actually does have several unique symptoms. For example, some patients never show the upper-respiratory symptoms or rash characteristic of other pneumonias; and more than half of the patients develop severe headache, confusion, and delirium—much rarer with "pneumonia." Interestingly, no one noticed these differences until it had been decided that Legionnaire's disease was indeed a new disease. All eyes were looking at the commonalities; unusual features were dismissed as idiosyncrasies. It took the outbreak in Philadelphia to highlight an unusual pattern of occurrence (an epidemic). Only then did investigators start seeing different features as relevant and come to identify a new disease based on a new bacterium.

In his book on AIDS, however, Victor Gong raises an important question about these apparently out-of-the-blue diseases. "A decade ago," he writes, "Legionnaire's disease, toxic shock syndrome, and AIDS were unknown. A question immediately comes to mind: Are we giving old diseases new names or suddenly confronting an array of microbes never encountered before?"[43] Some people have hypothesized, for example, that the AIDS virus arose years ago in Africa and may have been brought to other countries by immigrants or tourists. Alternatively, the virus might already have existed in a less lethal form and, over time, might have mutated into the variety we know today. Similar theories about syphilis have been suggested for years by historians.[44] In cases like these, the appearance of a new disease depends on such factors as technology or a changing worldview.

As a matter of fact, the chances are very high that even if the

AIDS virus had existed before the late 1970s, we wouldn't have had the knowledge or tools to discover it. As Secretary of Health and Human Services Margaret Heckler put it:

> Imagine the dilemma if AIDS had been identified in 1961 instead of 1981. A medical generation ago, we knew virtually nothing about monoclonal antibody testing as applied to research into B and T lymphocytes. The existence of interleukin II had not even been suspected. We had not discovered the enzyme, reverse transcriptase, which is produced by retroviruses and allows them to produce a DNA analogue of their RNA. Nor did we know about restriction endonuclease mapping of complex nucleic acid specimens, a procedure used to characterize the genes of viruses. Our base, our foundation of knowledge, was woefully lacking in pivotal blocks of scientific information.[45]

In fact, the AIDS virus might very well have been around—if not for centuries, at least for several decades—before it was recognized. As early as 1960 a group of doctors described a patient in the *Lancet* who had cytomegalic inclusion disease together with *Pneumocystis carinii* infection. The patient, who was not married, had been been previously ill, had traveled abroad while serving in the navy (from 1955 to 1957), and had numerous symptoms that suggested a decreased resistance to infection. When this man was admitted to the Manchester Royal Infirmary in April 1959, however, no one could name his disease, which quickly progressed and resulted in death by September. In 1983 the same group of doctors who had originally described this case wondered: "Perhaps AIDS is not a new disease; rare examples may in the past have masqueraded under various diagnoses."[46]

The case of Robert R., a fifteen-year-old St. Louis boy who died mysteriously in 1969, makes this hypothesis even more likely. For no apparent reason, this boy developed swollen lymph nodes in his neck as well as swelling of the legs, lower torso, and genitalia. Doctors surgically drained his lymph nodes, but after fifteen months he had not improved at all; in fact, he had lost weight and developed a severe *Chlamydia* infection (a genus of sexually transmitted bacteria that frequently infects gay men). Despite antibiotic treatment, he died after a bout with bronchial pneumonia, and an autopsy revealed that Robert R. also suffered from Kaposi's sarcoma. Looking back on this case in 1984, Robert R.'s doctors were struck by how these clues suggested

AIDS. Most convincing, however, was a follow-up study of Robert R.'s tissues (fortuitously saved), which revealed the presence of the AIDS virus.[47]

Thus, it is important to recognize that a brand-new virus may be causing illness for years before anyone identifies that illness as a new disease. In fact, what seem to be new diseases may sometimes turn out to be nothing more than *newly recognized* diseases.[48]

CHAPTER 8

How Diseases Change Their Meanings

The fact that diseases can come and go helps explain why some people can't find names for their illnesses: they may simply be living their lives at a time when their condition is between names. On the other hand, even if you happen to have a disease with a name, the meaning of that name is not always so clear. Not only can a different meaning result in different connotations about the nature of your illness, but in some cases it can allow certain people to regard what you thought was a full-fledged disease to be no disease at all.

▲ LYDIA'S DIFFERENT DIABETES

At forty years of age, Lydia found out that she had type II diabetes. Though naturally saddened at the time, she was mainly relieved: although she would have to lose weight and cut down on sweets, she felt better knowing that all her bothersome thirst and itching would end and that she wouldn't drop dead the next day. And in fact, today, a couple of years later, Lydia usually feels alert and healthy, and when she tells her close friends about her illness, she merely says that she has "diabetes," not wanting to go into technical detail.

Unfortunately, though, Lydia has very concerned friends; and every time one of them hears something about diabetes, Lydia's phone rings, usually with useless information. For example, Bella, Lydia's next-door neighbor, once called when she heard that genetic engineering firms were going to start producing insulin at a much lower cost. Lydia thanked her but said that so long as she keeps her weight down, she functions like a healthy person. Unlike people with uncontrolled diabetes, she tells her friend, she never requires insulin at all (despite this reassurance, Bella keeps a Hershey bar on hand, just in case Lydia is ever over having coffee and has an insulin reaction).

Worse, when the local university began running trials on a new drug to suppress antibodies against insulin, they ran an advertisement in the neighborhood paper asking for volunteers, specifically persons with type I diabetes. They only wanted people with this form of diabetes in which the body apparently builds up antibodies against its own insulin-producing cells, thus impairing sugar regulation. This is not at all true in people like Lydia with type II diabetes. Even so, Lydia received three calls that day from friends who wondered if she would consider volunteering: "As long as you have to be sick," said one, "you might as well help science." Gritting her teeth, Lydia explained that the volunteers would probably be children with type I diabetes.

▲ CONSUMING CONSUMPTION

Throughout medical history, the meaning of a disease has changed faster than its name. Thus, even though two people may use the same term, the actual condition described may be entirely different. The old disease "consumption" is worth examining in some detail here, since medical historians, most notably Lester S. King, have already elucidated the subtle and not-so-subtle shifts in meaning that occurred as technology and values changed.[1] These shifts in a term's meaning are by no means unique to medical history or to consumption, of course, but focusing the lenses of hindsight on earlier beliefs may help clarify processes that continue today.

Consumption was a disease your great-grandmother might have dreaded, but today you won't even find it listed in a medical text. This is not because consumption has been wiped from the face of the earth; it is simply hiding under the name of tuberculosis. Only for the past hundred years or so, however, have the words "consumption" and "tuberculosis" meant the same thing—making it redundant to talk of consumption, since it is equivalent to the very distinct disease tuberculosis.

In today's medical texts, "tuberculosis" means an infectious disease caused by a species of the bacillus *Mycobacterium*. Various organs react to these tubercle bacilli or their products by forming small rounded nodules called "tubercles." When cells that are infected with the bacillus die, they also emit a characteristic cheeselike substance; this emission process is called "caseation." Although the tuberculosis bacteria usually infect the lungs, they can spread through the bloodstream to infect other organs, including the heart, the intestines, the liver, the bones, the joints, and the lymph nodes.

Tubercles and caseation aren't visible to the naked eye, of course, and people with tuberculosis may experience no symptoms for many years. Others may gradually notice that they are developing symptoms such as fever, malaise, or weight loss (the term "consumption" originally referred to the "wasting away" of the body in these people). But in more severe cases, the disease can be brutal: patients may cough up sputum or blood, they may have trouble breathing, their chest walls may ache, and their lungs may fail altogether. In the nineteenth century, in fact—before effective drug therapy was developed—tuberculosis was a major public health problem known as the "white plague."

The disease we now know as tuberculosis has probably haunted mankind for more than two thousand years.[2] People of many times and cultures were probably infected by tubercle bacilli, and they probably developed the symptoms familiar to us today. But only for the past hundred years or so have doctors said that these people all had "tuberculosis" or "consumption." In fact, only for the past hundred years have doctors recognized that all people infected with these tubercle bacteria and showing these symptoms had one and the same disease; before then, some of these people were said to have "consumption" (or "phthisis" or "tabes"), some "scrofula," some "pneumonia," some "catarrh," and some nothing at all. Only with the discovery of the tubercle bacillus could doctors link these many different names together as examples of one disease: tuberculosis.

If you understand that the modern definition of tuberculosis depends on a lot of observations and knowledge that wouldn't have been available to the ancient Greeks or even to nineteenth-century doctors, you'll begin to understand why the older name "consumption" could change its meaning so many times. To define tuberculosis as we do today, doctors have had to obtain the tissues of people who died from tuberculosis, to characterize the tubercles with powerful microscopes and X-rays, and to analyze the type of bacteria they found.

Without microscopes, X-rays, dissection skills, or knowledge of microorganisms, doctors could rely only on their five senses to define their patients' illness. All they had to go by were symptoms. If someone came in with a cough and weight loss, then, a doctor might describe the disease as consumption—the patient was being "consumed," so to speak. Other doctors would see emaciated patients who were also spitting up pus or blood, and they, too, labeled the disease consumption (or "phthisis," the Greek word for "consumption").

For a long time, then, the term "consumption" was quite literal: it had nothing to do with tubercles on the lungs or a tubercle bacillus in the tissues; it simply described a set of symptoms. Without modern laboratory techniques, doctors could hardly have been expected to connect these symptoms with the tubercles and the tubercle bacillus. Nor could they be expected to know that the disease was associated with a microscopic organism, or be expected not to link it to heredity or even to frivolous or foolish behavior—such as tobacco-chewing, excessive drinking, and careless exposure to the elements.

As a result, for many centuries doctors mixed patients who today would be said to have tuberculosis with patients who had coughed and spit up pus and mucus but who really had different lung conditions—conditions not caused by the tubercle bacillus but which could produce the same symptoms. Because no one knew about tubercles or bacteria, and because no one knew how to distinguish pus from mucus or from other substances, there was no reason not to regard these diseases as consumption; they looked identical. So, for a while the term "consumption," or "phthisis," meant not only the very specific condition we today call tuberculosis, but also conditions such as bronchitis or emphysema or gangrene of the lungs.[3]

Over the years, scientists and doctors picked out certain symptoms they saw occurring together and called them consumption or different kinds of consumption. One observer found twenty varieties, for example, while another found fourteen. Again, without modern technology, these contradictory findings are understandable; and, as we have seen, as late as the eighteenth century, doctors were still relying mainly on observable signs and symptoms to define diseases. One seventeenth-century English doctor, Richard Morton (1635–1698), maintained that people with consumption shared three traits: 1) they showed signs of wasting throughout the entire body; 2) they had daily fevers with profound sweating, chills, and flushed countenance; and 3) they had lesions or "swellings" on the lungs that eventually filled dry coughs with pus.[4]

Morton's recognition of these lesions—known today as tubercles—marked a real change in the meaning of consumption. At least in theory, this seventeenth-century doctor had come up with a way to distinguish consumption from other diseases that produced similar symptoms: he connected it with a characteristic lesion in the body. Although in practice the technology of the time made it quite difficult to distinguish these particular swellings from other lesions, Morton's consumption was a more specific condition than the consumption of the ancients.

Morton's consumption differed from later consumption, however. For example, it did not include infection of organs besides the lungs. Today we know that when a certain species of tubercle bacillus (actually the bovine species, which generally prefers cattle to humans) infects the lymph nodes, a condition known as scrofula develops: lymph glands, especially in the neck, swell markedly, and often other lesions appear on the skin and mucous membranes. Scrofula develops principally (but not always) in children and, unlike consumption of the lungs, rarely produces emaciation, cough, or fever.

Now try to imagine a seventeenth-century doctor looking at a child with chronically swollen lymph glands in his neck. The child's symptoms looked very different from the symptoms of an adult with consumption—and symptoms were all the doctor had to go by. Seventeenth-century doctors knew nothing about bacilli and had no way of knowing that both scrofula and consumption involved tubercles caused by a tubercle bacillus; to them, scrofula looked like an entirely separate disease, not another variety of consumption.[5]

When you look closely, it's easy to understand how this "mistake" arose. Scrofula did indeed look like an entirely separate disease; unlike consumption, it mainly affected children, and, unlike consumption, it rarely produced fever, cough, or emaciation. Given this different group of people affected and these different symptoms, it is easy to see why doctors would separate the two conditions.[6] The only reason for seventeenth-century doctors even to suspect a connection of any kind was that, very often, children who had had scrofula would later develop true consumption of the lungs. Some of these doctors, including Morton, therefore speculated that scrofula and consumption were not entirely separate diseases but were actually two phases of the same disease. The modern answer, however, could only come when someone was able to prove that both conditions involved the same kind of tubercles and could then differentiate the species of bacillus causing the tubercles of scrofula from the species causing the tubercles of human tuberculosis. This sort of proof was impossible in seventeenth-century England.

Only later did researchers realize that the symptoms they called scrofula actually represented several quite distinct conditions. Often they represented a form of tuberculosis or consumption in which one species of tuberculosis bacterium had infected the lymph glands; at other times, they represented other diseases which had nothing to do with tuberculosis but which produced symptoms that looked like true scrofula.[7]

It wasn't until the mid-nineteenth century that anyone seriously proposed that consumption and scrofula had a related origin. By this time, a few investigators posited that some definite constitution of the blood—the essence of consumption—somehow caused both the swelling of the lymph glands associated with scrofula as well as the emaciation and coughing associated with consumption. Even then, however, current knowledge failed to support such a hypothesis. When you think about it, in fact, before the discovery of a specific bacterium, such a vague explanation sounds a lot more mystical than the old view in which doctors took what they saw to be separate diseases and let it go at that.

Later generations defined "consumption" according to the medical thinking and technology of their day—many times including conditions we now consider to be forms of different diseases; at other times, excluding conditions we now consider to be part of tuberculosis. The term took on its modern meaning only when Robert Koch (1843–1910) discovered the tubercle bacillus in 1881 and showed that it produced the symptoms of consumption.[8] In 1865 the French investigator Jean-Antoine Villemin (1827–1892) had proved that consumption was an infectious disease—both the caseous matter and the tubercles could be inoculated from one animal into another and produce the symptoms of consumption.[9] Now, Koch's discovery completed the proof by showing that the one thing all patients with consumption had in common was not a particular symptom (such as weight loss or lung failure) or a particular tissue lesion (such as a tubercle), but the presence of the tubercle bacillus. Suddenly it made sense how there could be many different forms of one disease: they all had the same origin.

As later investigators refined Koch's conclusion, they were able to show tubercle bacilli not only in the various tubercular tissues of the lungs, but in the tissues of other infected organs. All this meant that many of the disease names that had been assigned to each of these conditions—such as many different types of pneumonia and "catarrh"—suddenly disappeared or changed their meanings. All of these conditions were at last united into a single, specific infectious disease with a uniform etiology.[10]

In short, the discovery of a bacillus common to all people with consumption changed the meaning of consumption once again. The meaning expanded in the sense that the label "consumptive" now encompassed people previously thought to have catarrh or pneumonia. But the meaning also shrunk, in the sense that people previously thought to have consumption because they had abnormally shaped lung cells were now excluded if their symptoms arose from a condition linked to a lung cancer rather than to the tubercle bacillus.

▲ OUTGROWING A NAME

The story of consumption is hardly unique. As the physician and philosopher of medicine George L. Engel once argued, "Names for diseases often originated from the more obvious rather than from the more important characteristics of the condition or from some etiologic factor." For example, he continues, "pernicious anemia" is neither simply a disease of the blood, as "anemia" implies, nor is it any longer pernicious. The medical philosopher F. Kräupl Taylor likewise points out that the term "influenza" originally signified "the concept of some noxious 'influence' exerted by certain planetary constellations which were thought to cause seasonal epidemics of certain symptoms." He adds that the term "hysteria" formerly signified "a pathologically wandering womb" and that "rheumatism" once referred to the mucous "rheum" which emerged from the nose in a head cold and supposedly seeped into joints and muscles, making them swollen and painful.[11] Explaining that names of diseases generally reflect our knowledge of the condition at the time it is identified, Engel adds that while "our understanding of the processes involved is constantly changing, names are rarely changed, and they often continue to exert a weighty influence on the physician's concepts."[12]

Gout, for example, is a disease (actually a heterogeneous group of diseases) known since the beginnings of recorded medical history. Over time, though, the meaning of the term "gout" has become increasingly specific. Ancient Greek and Roman physicians described various conditions that involved this form of arthritis, calling it things like podagra (literally "foot seizure" or "foot grabber"), cheiragra ("hand seizure"), gonagra ("knee seizure"), or omagra ("shoulder seizure"), depending on which part of the body was affected. In the thirteenth century, the condition came to be known as "gout," a word derived from the Latin *gutta,* meaning "drop," for it was believed that the disease resulted from the dripping of bodily fluids—one of the four humors—into parts of the body where they didn't belong.

But what medieval physicians called "gout" was not the same thing as what we call "gout" today. Although it appears that earlier physicians distinguished podagra from other arthritic afflictions, doctors until at least the mid-sixteenth century, and probably much later, used the term "gout" to include people we now consider to be suffering from conditions such as rheumatic fever and rheumatoid arthritis. Throughout much of this time, gout was a rather fashionable ("in") disease, called the "disease of lords" and associated with a rich lifestyle, but it is now clear that many of the people believing themselves to have gout really had something less lordly. Only in the mid-nineteenth century did Sir Alfred Baring Garrod (1819–1907), known among historians as the "high priest of gout," show conclusively that gout, unlike all other forms of arthritis, was characterized by accumulations of uric acid in the blood serum and accumulations of sodium urate crystals in and around the afflicted joints.[13]

"Typhus" is another medical term that over the years has referred to a variety of conditions. Originally the term referred to a rather imprecise group of illnesses that, until the second third of the nineteenth century, included just about any state involving both fever and observable stupor. The term "typhus" transliterates the Greek word for "smoke" or "vapor," and until at least 1836 most doctors applied the term to any febrile patient who experienced exhaustion and a "cloudy sensorium"—without regard to other symptoms and, of course, without any knowledge that these same conditions could be accompanied by different internal lesions, evoked by different microbial organisms, or treatable with different drugs. Thus, a single term encompassed what today we would consider two separate diseases—typhoid fever and typhus—as well as apoplexy, influenza, and various forms of encephalitis and meningitis.

Today we think of typhus as a louse-borne infection produced by a group of microorganisms called rickettsia that share certain properties with bacteria as well as viruses. Patients experience prolonged high fever, intense headaches, and, almost always, a rash of small, pink flat spots that later become dark and partially raised. Even today, fatalities from typhus can be as high as 60 percent in older patients. In contrast, today's typhoid fever is an infectious bacterial disease caused by the bacillus *Salmonella typhi,* usually spread via contaminated food or water and marked by characteristic internal lesions, together with prolonged fever, exhaustion, abdominal pain, and, in about 10 percent of cases, a rose-colored rash. Before the advent of effective antibiotic therapy, 10 to 15 percent of afflicted patients died of the disease, but today prompt diagnosis and appropriate therapy can limit illness to a few days of fever and malaise.[14]

Until the middle of the eighteenth century, doctors called what we would now call either typhus or typhoid fever by many different names. As part of his pioneering nosological efforts, François Boissier de Sauvages is credited with first using the term "typhus" to designate a specific disease, and the term was generally adopted after Britain's influential William Cullen (1710–1790) took it up in 1772. Exactly what "typhus" meant, however, varied from one observer to the next. Often offering versions of Benjamin Rush's "one fever, one disease" theory, many leading medical thinkers in the next seventy-five years or so continued to see typhus not as a single, distinct disease but rather as an unspecific typhuslike (typhous or typhoid) state that could either "pass into" other diseases such as ones we might now call malaria or become a sort of intermediate disease with characteristics of both standard typhus and standard malaria. By distinguishing fever states not by symptoms but by principal organ involved, moreover, the early public health leader Thomas Southwood Smith (1788–1861) used the term "typhus" to include what we today would call purulent meningitis, tuberculous meningitis, influenza, typhoid fever, and cerebral infarctions.[15]

The first decades of the nineteenth century, however, saw new methodologies and investigative techniques in biochemistry, cell theory, anatomy, and physiology as well as new ways of thinking. With these innovations came accumulating evidence indicating that the term "typhus" referred not to one but to many distinct conditions. Careful observations of symptoms and epidemiology led investigators such as New England's Nathan Smith (1762–1829), the founder of Dartmouth Medical School, to conclude that the disease called "typhous fever" in America was a specific disease that spread from person to person and that, once acquired, would never strike again. But because Smith could offer no anatomical studies or even telltale symptoms to distinguish this fever from all others, his findings convinced very few of his peers. More convincing was the work of many French investigators, culminating in that of Pierre Louis (1787–1872) and Pierre-Fidèle Bretonneau (1771–1852), which correlated autopsy results with patient symptoms in order to determine that the disease they called "typhus" was characterized by ulcerations in a part of the small intestine. The French investigators called this specific disease "typhoid fever."[16]

One American greatly influenced by these findings was William Gerhard (1809–1872), who used techniques he had acquired as a student in Paris to show that the disease the French called typhoid fever was identical to the one the Americans called typhus—and, more important, that it was a disease distinct from the similar condition in which patients showed fever and stupor but showed no intestinal lesions. Two years later, Gerhard had a chance to study the two conditions simultaneously. An influx of Irish immigrants, who brought with them a "typhus" not previously recognized in the United States, came to Pennsylvania Hospital, where there were also many patients suffering from the "typhus" familiar to American doctors (the French typhoid fever). Gerhard, using clinical as well as pathological data, showed that despite the single name, "typhus" represented two distinct entities: one, our present-day typhoid fever, formerly called typhus mitior, was prevalent in France and the United States; the other, today's typhus, formerly called typhus gravior, ship fever, jail fever, camp fever, and petechial or spotted fever, was more prevalent in Great Britain and Ireland. While typhoid fever typically involved internal lesions and usually spread sporadically, typhus typically involved a specific skin rash and spread epidemically. Gerhard realized that what British investigators had to say about their "typhus" had little to do with what French and American investigators had to say about their disease of the same name.[17]

Whether typhus and typhoid fever were really separate diseases worthy of separate terms, however, or whether they were simply variations of a single disease, remained unclear. Elisha Bartlett (1804–1855), in his highly influential text on fevers (first published in 1843, expanded in 1847), supported Gerhard's findings and emphasized the difference between individual symptoms—the typhoid state—and the actual disease typhoid fever. Just because two patients shared a few symptoms—but not an overall pattern—did not mean they shared the same disease. Austin Flint, the prominent New York City clinician and educator who would later become a president of the American Medical Association, made similar arguments after he found that a mysterious epidemic in Buffalo, New York, in 1843 was the same typhoid fever known in New England and investigated by Pierre Louis in Paris. Many physicians, still mired in eighteenth-century thought, including Benjamin Rush's views, could read Bartlett's book and hear about Flint's studies without picking up this point, and there were still enough doctors who defined diseases solely on the basis of symptoms to leave the exact definition of typhus unclear.[18]

Only a few decades later, though, bacteriological research showed that the two conditions had different causes, and the medical profession as a whole accepted that typhus and typhoid fever were more than variants of a single entity. In 1880 the bacteriologist Karl Joseph Eberth of Zurich used new methods of staining to discover a specific bacillus associated with typhoid fever; the renowned German investigator Robert Koch confirmed Eberth's findings in 1881. After George Gaffky succeeded in growing this microorganism in pure culture (1884), it became generally accepted as the cause of typhoid fever, although proof was not rigorously completed until 1911. By the close of the nineteenth century, doctors had two different clinical-anatomical patterns differentiating typhoid fever from typhus, and, if there were ever any confusion, the association of the causal microorganism resolved any disputes.[19]

Typhus thus acquired a much sharper, more precise definition than it had when Cullen had first used the term nearly a hundred and fifty years earlier. The separate term "typhoid fever," however, still required some fine-tuning; for it later turned out that this term included not only today's typhoid fever, associated with *S. typhi,* but other infections that had symptoms similar to those of typhoid fever but which were caused by other species of *Salmonella.*

This same kind of change in the meaning of a disease term can occur over much shorter periods of time. Take endometriosis, for example. While studying this disease, doctors noticed another affliction of women which they called adenomyosis. In this condition, a benign tumor made up of muscle and resembling a gland appears on the inner muscular wall of the uterus. Because adenomyosis takes place strictly *inside* the uterus, most researchers and doctors considered it to be a distinct disease from endometriosis.[20]

And, in fact, they had a point. As many doctors still argue, endometriosis and adenomyosis feel different to the patient, occur in different types of women, and require different treatments. Yet, many prominent obstetricians and gynecologists respond that although these points are true enough, adenomyosis is a just a form of endometriosis—not an entirely separate disease. To bolster their point, they cite recent research that shows how both conditions involve the same basic process: namely, endometrial tissue gone astray (in adenomyosis, this tissue implants itself in tumors; in endometriosis, it implants itself in external organs). Thus, it is argued, they have enough in common to be considered the same disease, despite the differences. If these doctors win the day using these new findings, endometriosis will indeed transform its meaning—what endometriosis meant in 1920 will not be the same as what it means in the 1990s.

▲ PLAYING WITH STATISTICS

Perhaps even more strikingly, the meaning of AIDS seems to change every time you turn around—and, as the meaning changes, so do the chances of people with the disease. Right now, doctors are starting to consider anyone who carries the AIDS virus, whether or not they show any symptoms, as having the immunodeficiency disease. But as noted in earlier chapters, AIDS was until recently defined by specific opportunistic infections, rather than by the presence of the virus alone. Therefore, many people who shared certain problems with AIDS patients—such as diseased lymph nodes, low platelet levels, and various tumors—were considered to have a different condition called AIDS-related complex, or ARC.[21] These people had the AIDS virus in their blood and some even died of their condition, but until 1988 they didn't meet the exact criteria for AIDS.

In March 1987, 30,000 people had AIDS, but 150,000 to 300,000 had ARC. One of the reasons the range estimated for ARC was so broad is that, unlike AIDS, this condition had no standard definition—and since many of the symptoms occurred with other infections, different doctors assigned different labels to what indeed could have been the same condition. In fact, ARC was more a collection of symptoms than it was a specific disease. Moreover, it was defined largely by exclusion: when other causes for the symptoms had been ruled out, doctors concluded that the person must have ARC. Consequently, noted the epidemiologist Peter Drotman, "The diagnosis will vary, depending on what an individual physician's view is." One of the reasons the debate about AIDS and ARC was so strong, in fact, is that AIDS itself was (and still is) a new and rather unestablished disease; thus, its boundaries were particularly unclear.

In 1987, however, there was more and more talk about expanding the definition of AIDS to include ARC, as well as certain other conditions that seemed to be associated with the AIDS virus. By 1988 the change had been made. What is particularly interesting here is that along with the change in the definition came an immediate change in all the "facts" about what happens in AIDS. In 1985, for example, the Centers for Disease Control reported that 58 percent of the AIDS cases reported so far had resulted in death. But only one in ten ARC cases had resulted in death.[22] So, by adding the ARC cases to the AIDS cases, more people were reported to have "AIDS," but fewer of them were expected to die of it. In other words, the number of victims had increased, but their chances for survival had improved. Having AIDS now meant something very different.[23]

The converse point might be made about "Alzheimer's disease," a condition of mental deterioration in middle-aged and elderly people, which, as with many other nameless and shifting diseases, appears more and more to be not one specific disease but rather a generic term embracing a number of different conditions. Whether one disease or many, doctors reported a tenfold rise in deaths from Alzheimer's disease during the 1980s. And yet, there is some statistical evidence that this increased risk of dying may be related to nothing more than physicians' greater awareness of Alzheimer's disease, rather than to a sharp rise in the number of people contracting it or a shift in the seriousness of the condition. By calling things "Alzheimer's" which were previously diagnosed as other conditions, we may well have changed Alzheimer's disease from a relatively rare disease to a relatively common and dangerous one.[24]

Simply realizing this relationship between the meaning of a given disease name and the statistical probabilities attached to that name could not only reduce confusion, but also alleviate much unnecessary grief and fear. If your family history indicates that great-great-grandmother Agatha died of cancer, for example, you may fear a similar fate (especially after all those years of smoking). But what Grandma called "cancer" may have been an entirely different disease than what we call "cancer" today. In the early nineteenth century, the term meant a certain kind of painful and often fatal external growth. For most of the medical profession until the middle of the nineteenth century, "cancer" was a generic term that included tumors, cysts, and inflammatory masses.[25] And in the eyes of the average practitioner, this "cancer," which was known at times to become painful and even fatal, had cures, such as mixing "corrosive sublimate" (a mercurial preparation) into strong liquor and rubbing it on the skin to destroy the cancer.[26] Unfortunately, a splash of medicated whisky is not so effective in treating the variety of conditions we call "cancer" today.

▲ SPEAKING LIKE A DOCTOR

The meaning of a disease name can change according to who is doing the talking. Because they are using the same terms, for example, doctors and patients often think they are talking about the same things. But as the Gershwin song put it, "It ain't necessarily so." Let's say a patient goes to a doctor and says that she has "rheumatism." The patient means that she has the symptoms of rheumatoid arthritis: her joints feel stiff, painful, and weak and may look deformed. To the doctor, though, the term "rheumatism" means that the patient could have any one of many conditions, not just stiff joints; for the doctor, "rheumatism" is just a shorthand term for hundreds of rheumatic diseases. Rheumatoid arthritis is one of these diseases, which also include such diverse conditions as ankylosing spondylitis, fibrositis, tendonitis, carpal tunnel syndrome, gout, systemic lupus erythematosis, and many others.[27] In fact, any inflamed, degenerated, or metabolically disturbed connective tissues—including those in the heart and the brain—may be called "rheumatic."

The patient says "rheumatism," then, and so does the doctor, and both mistakenly think they are talking about the same thing.[28] Similar misunderstandings are common when patients come in claiming that they have "hypertension," "biliousness," "indigestion," "eye strain," and "fibrositis."[29] These words all have meanings to the layperson that are very different from the technical meanings they represent for the doctor. None of this would be so important if doctors simply realized that patients were describing something different, but, unfortunately, many doctors unconsciously assume that they speak the same language as the patient. If a patient describes her husband as "bilious," she may mean that the man has been in a foul temper or that he has looked rather pale lately; most doctors, however, would immediately assume that the man has been experiencing nausea, abdominal discomfort, frequent belching, and lack of appetite. As a result, a doctor may be writing prescriptions for antacids and scheduling blood tests when, in fact, the man may just need a vacation.

It is easy to understand how this could happen. Doctors, after all, assume that their patients share a language and culture with them. This assumption of commonality means they may let down their guard and unconsciously assume that they and their patients are speaking the same language, just as many Americans do when they visit England. But any American who compliments his British hostess on her lovely "pants" or mentions that he feels a bit "sick," only to be whisked off to the W.C., will soon realize that similar cultures can use words in very different ways.[30]

▲ THE LANGUAGE OF THE LABORATORY

Sometimes two different groups of investigators will speak different languages as well and consequently skew medical research. A difference in vocabulary can sometimes explain why two groups of respectable researchers can come up with remarkably diverse results.[31] Consider, for example, "Bonnie," an investigator testing out a new cure for dysmenorrhea (severe menstrual cramps). A few years earlier, Bonnie had found high levels of a hormonelike chemical called prostaglandin in the blood of women who suffer from these cramps, and this particular chemical had been known to cause cramps and contractions in other situations. The term "dysmenorrhea" suddenly was on the verge of acquiring a new meaning: not only did it imply severe menstrual cramps, but now these cramps had to be associated with a specific biochemical imbalance. Bonnie hypothesized that by injecting a drug which inhibits these cramp-causing prostaglandins, she might be able to curtail dysmenorrhea. So she found fifty volunteers—women with severe menstrual cramps—and she instructed each to take a dose of an antiprostaglandin drug monthly. After three months, she found, cramps had diminished significantly for most of these women, and she concluded that she had a new cure.

So far so good. But when Bonnie's competitor "Fred" tried to replicate the experiment, he found that while cramps diminished for some of his patients, others felt no change, and still others developed worse pains. From a statistical perspective, Fred knew that this meant the new drug was ineffective as a cure for dysmenorrhea. He privately concluded that Bonnie was a charlatan, trying to make a name for herself, renew her grant money, and, above all, prove her "feminist" point that dysmenorrhea was a physiological problem, curable with medicine, and not "all in the head" as gynecologists had been claiming for years.

The truth, however, was that both investigators had conducted valid studies. The problem had to do with the label "dysmenorrhea." Whereas most of Bonnie's patients had dysmenorrhea owing to high levels of prostaglandins—the newer meaning of the term—many of Fred's did not. Some of the women he studied had cramps owing to pelvic adhesions, endometriosis, and fibroid tumors—*not* because of excess prostaglandins—and others had psychological difficulties that caused them to exaggerate their pain. The result was that a drug which inhibited prostaglandin had absolutely no effect on their cramps. Because Fred had simply equated the name "dysmenorrhea" with "menstrual cramping," he concluded that the new drug did not work at all.

The lesson seems simple enough: investigators must be careful to separate diseases properly; then patients will receive appropriate treatment, and investigations will be carried out meaningfully. At many points in time, however, there are no uniform criteria available for separating one disease from the next. Only hindsight makes Bonnie and Fred's particular case so clear. Think of it this way: before the new drugs had been vindicated as an effective therapy, there was no proof that excess prostaglandin was a meaningful way to separate some women with dysmenorrhea from other women with the same symptoms. All that doctors knew was that a group of women suffered from severe menstrual cramps; therefore, most doctors cared for all women with dysmenorrhea by prescribing medicines to relieve the pain. Only when further research showed that a specific treatment worked well for some of these women and not for others did prostaglandin levels become a relevant way to divide up this "disease." Thus, while Fred and Bonnie's experiments were in progress, it was still completely appropriate to consider "dysmenorrhea" to be one phenomenon, a phenomenon synonymous with "menstrual cramps."

The case of Fred and Bonnie is hypothetical, of course, but similar scenarios occur every day. For example, as Dr. James Alexander Hamilton, an authority on puerperal mental illness, has noted, psychiatrists in one study concluded that about one out of every two thousand mothers develops postpartum depression. Their methodology was straightforward. Investigators noted that after about one of every one thousand births, the mother needed to be hospitalized for mental illness. They then found that about half of these women were classified as having the disease "depression." Therefore, they concluded that only one of every two thousand births results in a mother with postpartum depression—not a very high incidence. This method seemed to make sense. Classically, "depression" has been applied to psychiatric patients who also happened to be depressed. But couldn't women show signs of depression following childbirth without being admitted to a mental hospital? Other investigators suspected that they could, Hamilton explains, and therefore looked for depressive symptoms in all mothers—not just in mothers already confined to psychiatric hospitals.

For this second group of investigators, "depression" had a totally different meaning: it was not a psychiatric illness, but a symptom of any one of several different illnesses. And so, when this group of sixty-five general practitioners wanted to know how commonly postpartum depression occurred, they looked at the reactions of 618 mothers who had recently given birth at a maternity hospital or clinic. The 618 women were examined by means of an interview, test, or question-naire to see whether they were "depressed." Again, in this case, "depression" was not a disease but a symptom. To be called "depressed," the women did not have to have problems severe enough to warrant psychiatric hospitalization; they simply had to feel depressed. Not surprisingly, then, these general practitioners found that the first study had grossly underestimated the frequency of postpartum depression. In fact, they (as well as other groups) found that 10 percent (that's *two hundred* out of every two thousand, not *one* out of two thousand) had enough depressive symptoms three months after childbirth to be called "depressed."[32]

This sort of confusion over meaning is especially common for nameless diseases, which have no clear-cut definitions in the first place. One of the reasons why some authorities can proclaim that dyslexia affects as many as 15 percent of children while other studies claim that only 3.5 percent of school-age children are affected is that not everyone agrees on the exact boundaries for a definition of dyslexia or on its pathophysiological origins. The fact that many people use terms such as "hyperactivity" and "learning disorder" synonymously with "dyslexia" may partially explain why they find more people with dyslexia than do those people who limit their definition to specific reading problems. Some authorities have suggested distinguishing the reading problems from the associated symptoms; the first would be called "dyslexia-pure" (just a reading disorder), and the second would be called "dyslexia-plus" (a reading disorder along with other behavioral traits such as hyperactivity, math difficulties, and lack of coordination). If investigators would limit their investigations to "dyslexia-pure" (as some do), perhaps some of the discrepancies would disappear.

Similar problems can result when different names have the same or nearly the same meaning. Sometimes, for example, various researchers (often working in different countries) will use different names for what is really best thought of as the same entity. Investigators worldwide now believe, for example, that various forms of "chronic fatigue syndrome" can result months or years after a viral infection or other trauma. The names for these forms vary from country to country and even from lab to lab, but debilitating fatigue and other associated symptoms characterize them all. Thus, while journals in Great Britain, Canada, Australia, South Africa, and the Netherlands have recently been publishing many articles about a "postviral fatigue syndrome" and about "myalgic encephalomyelitis" (ME), which may well be the same disease, American journals have been publishing articles about a "chronic fatigue syndrome" (or, more recently, a "chronic fatigue immune dysfunction syndrome"). Meanwhile, other researchers are studying identical or related conditions that go under completely different names, including "idiopathic chronic fatigue," "myalgic syndrome," "epidemic neuromyasthenia," "Royal Free disease," "low natural-killer cell syndrome," "persistent myalgia following sore throat," "Otago mystery disease," "Icelandic disease," and just plain "chronic fatigue."

There may, of course, be real differences between each of these names. For example, ME sometimes seems to be associated with epidemic outbreaks, whereas chronic fatigue immune dysfunction syndrome does not. Nevertheless, all of these nameless diseases remain so poorly defined that the terms must inevitably overlap to some degree.[33] Given the inexact definition of most of these names, it is likely that many people today who have "chronic fatigue" without having any other symptoms are being told they have one of these diseases or syndromes. It is also likely that some people categorized as having "chronic fatigue immune dysfunction syndrome" may actually turn out to have one of the other chronic fatigue syndromes, a mental disorder, or one of several as-yet-undefined conditions.

To understand the impact of this confusion on research, consider the following hypothetical possibility. Say that both America's "chronic fatigue immune dysfunction syndrome" and Great Britain's "ME" are really catchall terms, each of which includes different proportions of patients who have chronic fatigue linked to the Epstein-Barr virus, to the Coxsackie B virus, to a herpes virus, to retrovirus-like sequences and serum reactivity, to allergy, or to no known factor. Now say that following a short viral illness, you experience chronic fatigue after exercise, aching muscles, and frequent depression. If you live in Cleveland, Ohio, and meet up with a doctor who "believes" in such diseases, you might well be diagnosed as having "chronic fatigue immune dysfunction syndrome." On the other hand, if you live in Leeds, England, you probably would be diagnosed as having "ME." What a pity, then, that even if British investigators come up with a therapy for "ME," your doctor in Cleveland would never think of trying it on you, for you have "chronic fatigue immune dysfunction syndrome."[34]

Likewise, these different names with similar meanings can confuse the results of medical research itself. Investigators undermine each other's efforts because a lab in England studying "ME" may not necessarily realize that its results can be compared with those of a lab in America studying "chronic fatigue immune dysfunction syndrome." It may not understand that at least some of the patients studied may indeed turn out to have the same disease. Nor do most researchers suspect that one of the reasons they have so much trouble isolating a specific virus for any of these syndromes is that they may be lumping together patients who would better be divided into several different groups, each associated with a unique virus or other etiological factor.

Of course, it is crucial to stress that despite this constant need for refinement, some sort of classification is essential in practicing medicine. We could endlessly separate one patient from the next on the basis of different characteristics (she has brown hair, he has a wart, and so on), but this would obviate lessons from experience. In other words, we benefit from generalizing, and in order to do so we have to find certain similarities; otherwise, every new illness has no precedent whatsoever, and all treatments degenerate into blind stabs. The challenge, however, is to find the *relevant* similarities. In the dysmenorrhea example, doctors before Bonnie's experiment may have known that some women with dysmenorrhea had excess prostaglandins, but they also knew that some of these women had red hair; just because there were different kinds of sufferers didn't mean these differences were relevant.

▲ THE NAME'S THE SAME, BUT . . .

With this background, Lydia's problems with her type II diabetes become understandable. The name "diabetes"—which once referred to a specific problem regulating blood sugar—today has several distinct meanings. Clearly, just saying you have "diabetes" is no longer enough: type I diabetes is very different from type II. As we have seen, moreover, diabetes is hardly unique; as scientists and doctors learn more, the meanings of many disease names change. As years pass, the same name may be used to describe very different kinds of illness, and, as Lydia's case shows, confusion, aggravation, and even misleading research can result when different people interpret a name to mean something it no longer means.

Since the term "diabetes" was first applied to patients some two thousand years ago, in fact, it has taken on a number of increasingly specific meanings. Originally the term, which came from the Greek word for "siphon," referred solely to a disease characterized by excess thirst and excess urination: patients with the disease seem to act like giant siphons, taking in huge quantities of water and then excreting them. Sometimes doctors also observed a sweet taste to the urine (tasting urine was a long-standing diagnostic test in prelaboratory days). Until the end of the eighteenth century, this "diabetes" was thought to result from some disorder of the kidneys or digestive system.

In the middle of the seventeenth century, however, the meaning of "diabetes" began to change when Thomas Willis (1621–1675) differentiated diabetes mellitus (the more common form of diabetes today) from diabetes insipidus, as did various other doctors for more than a century thereafter. Diabetes insipidus does not involve impaired sugar metabolism and, according to some historians, may have been the disease described as "diabetes" by some ancient authors. In 1856 the term "diabetes" grew even more specific when it was proved conclusively that the disease is characterized by high levels of sugar in the blood (hyperglycemia) as well as in the urine. Not until the late nineteenth century, though, did it become clear that diabetes stems from a disorder of the pancreas or that it is related to an internal secretion of the islets of Langerhans, which rest atop the pancreas. In fact, this connection was not fully accepted until 1922, when the Canadian investigators Frederick Grant Banting and Charles Herbert Best showed that a potent extract (today known as insulin) from these islets could reverse the metabolic changes of diabetes.

Researchers later found that other hormones besides insulin could produce a diabetic state, and they began to suspect that there might be different types of diabetes. Then, as people with diabetes began to live longer, researchers found that they had to associate the term with a group of complications involving the arteries, eyes, kidneys, and feet. Today, the term "diabetes" has become so precise that it refers not to one condition but, rather, to a heterogeneous group of disorders, each characterized by hyperglycemia but each also stemming from one of a variety of pathways, including a deficiency of the cells producing insulin, an excess of hormones that counteract insulin, or even as a result of an abnormal insulin molecule.[35]

What Lydia's friends don't understand, therefore, is that "diabetes" is not a very meaningful term anymore. This is not a problem of getting the wrong name. Lydia does have diabetes. But the meaning of the term "diabetes" has become diluted over the years: although once it very specifically singled out patients who had problems metabolizing sugar, it is now a generic term for a variety of conditions.[36] Today, a doctor cannot treat a patient properly if all she knows is that the patient has diabetes; she must decide whether her patient has type I, type II, or some other form of diabetes before she can prescribe the right kind of treatment and predict the patient's outcome. Similarly, researchers today must specify what type of diabetes they are studying; otherwise, results can be skewed. Because disease names are not fixed for all time and all circumstances, a name means nothing unless someone specifies what it implies then and there.

▲

The Courage to Admit Ignorance

The greater the ignorance the greater the dogmatism.
—Sir William Osler

Given the immense complexity of the human body, it's hardly surprising that there are still many aches, pains, and feelings that doctors can't fit into some cut-and-dried category known as "a disease." Despite powerful tools and thousands of years of study, we've only just begun to understand how the heart or the brain works, much less how each organ influences other organs or how the body's countless chemicals, cells, and molecules interact. Nor is medical science beyond its infancy in understanding how individual backgrounds—different genes, surroundings, microorganisms, traumas, toxins, foods, and even behaviors—affect the body. Certainly modern medical science can cite its triumphs, but so much is still unknown that it makes perfect sense why we have to keep revising the patterns we call diseases. Once you have a little sense of history, in fact, it's ludicrous to think that, in contrast to all of humankind, we the living just happen to have been born at the one time in history when medical science at last has all the answers. When you think of the complexity of the human being and then consider everything that theoretically could go wrong with any part of us, it's truly amazing that we've managed to pick out so many specific diseases that correspond to individual human complaints.

Such thoughts make it easier to accept the fact that not all complaints are going to find names. If doctors can't assign a disease name to your condition, after all, it simply means that, given current evidence, they have been unable to fit your particular set of symptoms and signs into a known pattern. It does not mean that you are crazy, the doctors stupid, the discomfort minor, or the consequences trivial. Being assigned a name is merely a convenience for those of us lucky enough to be living in a time and place where our particular set of symptoms fits. And even for the unlucky ones, this understanding in and of itself can help alleviate self-doubt in the face of skeptical physicians, friends, and family. Further solace can come from continuing to search even while accepting that there may never be an answer. Much of the fear and anguish associated with the lack of a name can be diminished if patients find a sympathetic practitioner (rather than running from one stranger to another), become their own medical detectives, learn how to communicate symptoms to physicians, accept treatment for symptoms while lacking a diagnosis, and, on occasion, consider psychological counseling or tests.[1]

Early in the present book, we met Joe, the man with the unnamed abdominal pains. As we saw, some doctors might have blamed him rather than admit ignorance. To comfort him, they could have said, "It's all in your head" or "I'll run some more tests" or "It may be gastroenteritis. Try these pills [which turn out to be placebos]." Instead, however, Joe found a doctor who told him the truth. This doctor told Joe that he was merely unlucky—unlucky to be living in a culture that does not, or cannot, fit his particular symptoms into a pattern called a disease.

This truth does not make Joe any less ill. He still suffers from stomach upset, whether or not he is labeled as having a "duodenal ulcer," just as a woman feels the pain whether or not her cramps are called "dysmenorrhea" or "imaginary." After all, a rose by any other name would still have nasty thorns. Nor does this truth stop the doctor from prescribing medication to relieve the symptoms. What it does do, however, is put an end to what for Joe could have been a long, futile, and expensive search.

Of course, if Joe hadn't been willing to accept this truth, the result might also have been a lost patient for the honest doctor. As we have seen, many people are so desperate for a name that they will grasp onto names prematurely, mistaking syndromes and symptoms for names, for example, particularly when those names are attached to "in" diseases. If we are going to expect doctors to be honest, we have to be able to accept an "I don't know."

Right now, unfortunately, far too many patients, who for good reasons want names for their complaints, are pressuring doctors to give them answers that simply don't exist. When the more timid among us don't get the answer, we may grumble behind the doctor's back. How often, for example, have you heard an ailing friend return from the doctor complaining, "Well, it could be a drug reaction or another infection, but it's probably just a virus"? Cynical sorts add, "As usual, they have no idea what's going on." Then these same patients will often go to another doctor and try again, indirectly punishing the first doctor who didn't know the answer and was brave enough to admit it. Eventually, most doctors learn (often unconsciously) that to keep their patients happy they shouldn't be totally honest. The more forceful patients don't waste much time teaching doctors this lesson: they demand answers directly, complaining and probing until at last their doctors break down and name the symptom as though it were a disease. Some doctors even name a possible disease, despite a lack of concrete evidence, just to keep the patient happy. In the long run, of course, misdiagnoses make no one very happy.

Note that I am not accusing doctors of malpractice; very little of this behavior is conscious. Furthermore, in many ways, doctors who act this way are simply doing what their patients ask them to do. We often accuse doctors of "acting like God," but the truth is that we often ask them to do so. However experienced or powerful we become, throughout life we all retain the need for a parental figure—a priest, a teacher, a psychologist, or a physician—who knows more than we do, who gives us hope that the utter ineptitude and ignorance we sense in ourselves is not all there is to the world. To some extent, in fact, medicine works *because* patients believe it works and *because* they believe doctors have some special knowledge. Placebos take advantage of this belief: we may take a pill that the doctor knows to have no recognized biochemical effects, and our symptoms will go away just because we are confident the pill will work. Similarly, sometimes just believing that the doctor is powerful and knowledgeable is enough to help us feel better.[2]

Over time, such expectations on the part of patients will inevitably take their toll on a doctor's ability to admit ignorance. As George Bernard Shaw observed in his preface to *The Doctor's Dilemma,*

> When you [the doctor] are so poor that you cannot afford
> to refuse eighteenpence from a man who is too poor to
> pay you any more, it is useless to tell him that what he
> or his sick child needs is not medicine, but more lei-
> sure, better clothes, better food, and a better drained
> and ventilated house. It is kinder to give him a bottle of
> something almost as cheap as water, and tell him to
> come again with another eighteenpence if it does not
> cure him.[3]

Likewise, it is kinder to give his illness a name, with its associated outcome and treatment, than to say "I don't know" and leave him as scared
and helpless as ever.

Understanding what it really means to have a disease can
change this unfortunate situation. For doctors, this understanding
means withstanding the pressure to give all desperate patients a name
for their complaint. For patients, it means learning to accept doctors
who are strong enough to withstand the pressure and say, "Yes, you're
ill, but there's no known name for your disease." It also means that doctors will have to withstand the pressure to fit all conditions into pre-
established reimbursement categories and that researchers will have to
withstand the pressure to study an "in" disease before that disease has
been defined. We all have to learn to live with uncertainty, to view what
we know as incomplete and limited, and to use our knowledge to the
best of our abilities nonetheless.

Such conclusions may be hard to accept, given our great thirst
for certainty, especially in medicine. When it comes to our health, we
don't want to play guessing games; we want answers. And as patients,
we put tremendous pressure on doctors to give us those answers. If my
chest aches, I don't want to hear that there is a 25 percent chance that
I'm having a heart attack. I want to know whether or not I am having a
heart attack—period. Moreover, I want to know *now,* and I want to
know what I can do to get well—and I want to know that doing so *will*
make me well, not that there is a 63.5 percent chance that it will.

I have a feeling that this is a theme I will be preaching the rest of
my life, both to my readers and to myself. Yes, to myself too. Because
even though it may be easy to recognize uncertainty rationally, it is
hard to live with it. The other day, for example, my computer "got sick."
I was typing away merrily when suddenly the screen blacked out, and
the vents started puffing out gray smoke. Since I've become totally dependent on the machine these days, I immediately took it in for repairs;

several days later when it was discharged from the shop, the technician handed me the lethal bill. "What happened?" I asked.

"The power supply went," he replied.

"Why?" I went on. "Did it overheat, or was it just old, or what?"

"No. The power supply just does that sometimes."

"But can't I do something to prevent its happening in the future?"

"Buy a service contract," the man suggested, quite seriously.

The point is, I wanted an explanation so I could do something to prevent this inconvenient and expensive event from ever happening again. This is the same reason I want to know why a friend has had difficulty in labor—I would rather *blame* her, or blame her doctor, or blame her hospital, or else blame unique flaws in her life or physiology so that I can take steps to ensure this won't happen to me. I can't just stop at saying, "A terrible thing happened." Instead, I continue to search for the name of what went wrong so that I can reassure myself that the name and all it connotes will not apply to me or my life.

Unfortunately, however, although truth may be that simple and straightforward (after all, from an omniscient perspective, there is only one event happening, and only one outcome, and that event can be named), *knowledge* of truth is not. As we have seen throughout this book, new facts, new conditions keep impinging on our grand schemes, forcing us to reformulate what we once carved in stone. Although we must use our schemes "as if" they were carved in stone for as long as we can, we must always keep their fallibility safely tucked in the back of our minds and acknowledge that someday the stone may be erased. The history of medicine is littered with "certainty" undermined by experience and, later, through more experience, made "certain" again.

This is no last-minute hedging, no vague conclusion leaving the impression that "we don't know anything, and all is a jumble." No, it is, in fact, accepting this very indefiniteness which provides the answer; for as long as researchers remember that "a disease" is variable and therefore make sure they define their subject, they can avoid discrepancy. As long as doctors remember that known diseases are contingent on contemporary knowledge and societal values, they will be able to differentiate sickness from disease. As long as patients remember that a disease is a useful model but that not all illness can be fit into it, they will realize that they are not crazy or hypochondriacs. As Socrates knew well, there is no shame, but great wisdom, in admitting our ignorance.

Help
for Those
with
Nameless
Diseases

If you think you might be suffering from a nameless disease, the following organizations may be able to help. Devoted to educating the public about commonly overlooked, unrecognized, or misdiagnosed conditions, most of these groups issue regular newsletters and informational pamphlets, which can be obtained simply by writing to the addresses listed below (include a self-addressed stamped envelope with your request). Many of these associations also offer local support groups and helplines. Besides organizations that help victims of specific nameless diseases, the list includes a section of more general organizations that deal with such hard-to-identify conditions as "degenerative diseases" or "rare disorders." Also included are organizations for well-recognized conditions such as heart disease, arthritis, and cancer when those conditions represent classes of various disorders, some of which remain difficult to diagnose. In addition, there are brief descriptions for some lesser-known conditions not mentioned in the book.

▲ DISEASE-SPECIFIC ORGANIZATIONS

▲ AIDS AND AIDS-RELATED COMPLEX

Gay Men's Health Crisis
129 West 20th St.
New York, NY 10011
212-807-6655 (hotline)
212-807-6664

National AIDS Hotline
800-342-AIDS
800-344-SIDA (Spanish)
800-AIDS-TTY (for the hearing impaired)
[All hotlines are open seven days a week. The main hotline is available twenty-four hours a day, the Spanish-language hotline from 8:00 A.M. to 2:00 A.M. EST, and the hearing-impaired hotline (available only to those with a TTY machine) from 10:00 A.M. to 10:00 P.M. EST.]

National AIDS Network
2033 M St., N.W.
Suite 800
Washington, DC 20036
202-293-2437

National Association of People with AIDS
2025 I St., N.W.
Suite 415
Washington, DC 20006
202-429-2856

▲ ALOPECIA AREATA
[Alopecia areata is a rare, progressive condition that manifests itself in sudden hair loss, usually confined to the head and face, although the entire body may be involved. Because the disease is little understood, victims can experience social and occupational problems; they may also be denied insurance money for expensive, custom-made wigs because the disease is classified as a "cosmetic" problem.]

Help Alopecia International Research, Inc. (HAIR)
P.O. Box 691487
West Hollywood, CA 90069
213-851-5138

National Alopecia Areata Foundation
714 C Street
Suite 202
San Rafael, CA 94901
415-456-4644

▲ ALZHEIMER'S DISEASE

Alzheimer's Disease and Related Disorders Association
70 East Lake Street
Suite 600
Chicago, IL 60601
312-853-3060
800-621-0379 (hotline)

▲ ANOREXIA NERVOSA AND BULIMIA

Anorexia Nervosa and Related Eating Disorders
P.O. Box 5102
Eugene, OR 97405
503-344-1144

Bulimia/Anorexia Self-Help Hotline (BASH)
800-227-4785

National Anorexia Aid Society
5796 Karl Rd.
Columbus, OH 43229
614-436-1112

▲ ARTHRITIS

Arthritis Foundation
1314 Spring St., N.W.
Atlanta, GA 30309
404-872-7100

▲ ARTHROGRYPOSIS MULTIPLEX CONGENITA

[Arthrogryposis Multiplex Congenita, or AMC, is a birth defect involving limited joint movement. It is often confused with spina bifida, sacral agenesis, and damage to the brain and spinal column.]

Avenues, National Support Group for Arthrogryposis Multiplex Congenita
c/o Mary Ann Schmidt
P.O. Box 5192
Sonora, CA 95370
209-928-3688

▲ ATAXIA

[Ataxia is a hereditary disorder involving a progressively worse reeling, widestance gait caused by degeneration of nerves in the spinal cord and cerebellum. It may be confused with multiple sclerosis.]

National Ataxia Foundation
600 Twelve Oaks Center
15500 Wayzata Blvd.
Wayzata, MN 55391
612-473-7666

▲ AUTISM

Autism Society of America
1234 Massachusetts Ave., N.W.
Suite C-1017
Washington, DC 20005
202-783-0125

National Autism Hotline
Douglas Education Building
Tenth Ave. and Bruce St.
Huntington, WV 25701
304-525-8014

▲ CANCER

American Cancer Society
1599 Clifton Rd.
Atlanta, GA 30329
404-320-3333

Cancer Care, Inc.
1180 Avenue of the Americas
New York, NY 10036
212-221-3300

Cancer Federation, Inc.
11671 Sterling
Room J
Riverside, CA 92503
714-359-3794

Cancer Information Service
c/o National Cancer Institute
NIH Building 31
Room 10A24
Bethesda, MD 20892
800-4-CANCER (hotline)

Make Today Count
101½ South Union St.
Alexandria, VA 22314
703-548-9674

National Cancer Care Foundation
1180 Avenue of the Americas
New York, NY 10036
212-221-3300

▲ CELIAC SPRUE
[Celiac sprue is a genetic condition in which people cannot digest gluten—the protein portion of wheat, rye, and cereal grains. Symptoms can include abdominal bloating and discomfort, anemia, intestinal lesions, diarrhea, vomiting, weight loss, and skin disorders. Some patients exhibit only minor symptoms, however, making diagnosis difficult.]

Celiac Sprue Association/United States of America
2313 Rocklyn Dr.
Des Moines, IA 50322
515-270-9689

Gluten Intolerance Group of North America
P.O. Box 23053
Seattle, WA 98102
206-325-6980

▲ CEREBRAL PALSY

United Cerebral Palsy Associations
66 East 34th St.
New York, NY 10016
800-USA-1UCP

▲ CHRONIC FATIGUE IMMUNE DYSFUNCTION

Chronic Fatigue Immune Dysfunction Society Association
Community Health Services
1401 East Seventh St.
Charlotte, NC 28204
704-375-0172

Chronic Fatigue Syndrome Association
919 Scott Ave.
Kansas City, KS 66105
913-321-2278

Chronic Fatigue Syndrome Society
P.O. Box 230108
Portland, OR 97223
503-684-5261

▲ CROHN'S DISEASE

National Digestive Diseases Information Clearinghouse
Box NDDIC
Bethesda, MD 20892
301-468-6344

National Foundation of Ileitis and Colitis, Inc.
444 Park Ave. S.
New York, NY 10016
212-685-3440

▲ DEPRESSION

Depressives Anonymous: Recovery from Depression (DARFD)
329 East 62nd St.
New York, NY 10021
212-689-2600

National Depressive and Manic Depressive Association
P.O. Box 3395
Merchandise Mart
Chicago, IL 60654
312-939-2442

▲ DIABETES

American Diabetes Association, Inc.
1 West 48th St.
New York, NY 10020
212-947-9707
800-ADA-DISC (hotline)

▲ DYSLEXIA

National Institute of Dyslexia
3200 Woodbine St.
Chevy Chase, MD 20815
301-652-0942

The Orton Dyslexia Society
724 York Road
Baltimore, MD 21204
301-296-0232
800-ABCD-123 (hotline)

▲ ENDOMETRIOSIS

Endometriosis Society
65 Holmdene Ave.
Herne Hill
London SE24 9LD
England

U.S.-Canadian Endometriosis Association
8585 North 76th Pl.
Milwaukee, WI 53223
414-355-2200
800-992-ENDO (U.S.A.)
800-426-2END (Canada)

Victorian Endometriosis Association
c/o 37 Andrew Crescent
South Croydon, Victoria 3136
Australia

▲ EPILEPSY

Epilepsy Foundation of America
1828 L Street N.W.
Suite 406
Washington, DC 20036
800-EFA-3700
800-332-1000 (hotline)

▲ FIBROMYALGIA
[Fibromyalgia—also called fibrositis or chronic muscle pain syndrome—refers to any of several rheumatic disorders, all of which involve painful, tender, and stiff muscles and tendons, especially in the lower back, neck, shoulders, thorax, and thighs. It is often confused (and may overlap) with chronic fatigue immune dysfunction syndrome or dismissed as "all in your head."]

Arthritis Foundation
1314 Spring St., N.W.
Atlanta, GA 30309
404-872-7100

Arthritis Information Clearinghouse
Box AMS
Arlington, VA 22209
301-468-3235

Central Ohio Fibrositis Association
Riverside Methodist Hospital
North Medical Building
Suite 8
3545 Oletangy River Rd.
Columbus, OH 43214
614-262-8020

▲ FRAGILE X SYNDROME
[Fragile X syndrome is a genetic condition that can produce mental retardation in males and psychological disorders in females. Because it is hard to detect, this syndrome often goes undiagnosed.]

National Fragile X Foundation
P.O. Box 300233
Denver, CO 80203
800-835-2246

▲ HEART DISEASE

American Heart Association
7320 Greenville Ave.
Dallas, TX 75231
214-373-6300

Coronary Club
9500 Euclid Ave.
Cleveland, OH 44106
216-444-3690

Heartlife
340 Boulevard, N.E.
Atlanta, GA 30312
404-351-4515
800-241-6993

Mended Hearts
c/o American Heart Association
7320 Greenville Ave.
Dallas, TX 75231
214-706-1442

▲ HYPOGLYCEMIA

National Hypoglycemia Association
P.O. Box 120
Ridgewood, NJ 07451
201-670-1189

▲ INTERSTITIAL CYSTITIS

Interstitial Cystitis Association
P.O. Box 1553
Madison Square Station
New York, NY 10159
212-979-6057

▲ IRRITABLE BOWEL SYNDROME
[Irritable bowel syndrome, also known as spastic colon or mucous colitis, is an intestinal disorder characterized by abdominal pain, constipation, and diarrhea. Apparently a reaction to stress in susceptible individuals, IBS can be confused with numerous other conditions, including lactose intolerance, duodenal ulcer, allergies, thyroid problems, and various cancers.]

National Digestive Diseases Information Clearinghouse
Box NDDIC
Bethesda, MD 20892
301-468-6344

National Foundation of Ileitis and Colitis, Inc.
444 Park Ave., S.
New York, NY 10016
212-685-3440

▲ JOSEPH DISEASE
[Joseph disease, an inherited neurological disorder of the motor system, is often misdiagnosed as multiple sclerosis, Parkinson's disease, or spinocerebellar degeneration.]

International Joseph Disease Foundation
P.O. Box 2550
Livermore, CA 94550
(No phone number listed)

▲ LABYRINTHITIS

[Labyrinthitis is most accurately defined as an inflammation of the inner ear, but the term can also refer to a nameless disease characterized by repeated bouts of spontaneous dizziness, nausea, and vomiting, often after a trivial viral infection. Perhaps an aspect of the inner-ear diseases "vestibular neuronitis of Dix and Hallpike" or "recurrent peripheral vestibulopathy," labyrinthitis can be mistaken for brain tumors and various neurological and psychiatric problems.]

Dizziness and Balance Disorder Association
1015 Northwest 22nd Ave.
Portland, OR 97210
503-229-7348

▲ LEARNING DISABILITIES

Association for Children with Learning Disabilities
4156 Library Rd.
Pittsburgh, PA 15234
412-881-2253

▲ LUPUS ERYTHEMATOSUS

[Systemic lupus erythematosus, or SLE, is an inflammatory disorder of the connective tissue. Appearing predominantly in young women, symptoms and signs vary widely but can include joint pain, skin eruptions, lesions on areas exposed to light, fever, and a low white blood cell count. Although survival rates improve greatly if the disease is recognized and controlled, the early stages of SLE can be difficult to differentiate from other connective-tissue disorders such as rheumatoid arthritis. It is also commonly confused with multiple sclerosis and depression.]

The American Lupus Society
23751 Madison St.
Torrance, CA 90505
213-373-1335

L.E. Support Club
8039 Nora Ct.
North Charleston, SC 29418
803-764-1769

Lupus Foundation of America
1717 Massachusetts Ave., N.W.
Suite 203
Washington, DC 20036
202-328-4550
800-558-0121

Lupus Network
230 Ranch Dr.
Bridgeport, CT 06606
203-372-5795

▲ LYME DISEASE

The Lyme Borreliosis Foundation, Inc.
P.O. Box 462
Tolland, CT 06084
203-871-2900

▲ MARFAN SYNDROME
[Marfan syndrome is an inherited disorder of the connective tissue. Patients are taller than average for their age and family; fingers and toes are disproportionately long and thin; and often the sternum is deformed. There are also problems with the eyes, lungs, heart, and blood vessels, but because many patients have only a few symptoms, Marfan syndrome can easily be overlooked or confused with other diseases such as homocystinuria.]

National Marfan Foundation
382 Main St.
Port Washington, NY 11050
516-883-8712

▲ MEIGE'S SYNDROME
[Meige's syndrome consists of involuntary muscle spasms of the eyes, lower face, mouth, tongue, throat, and respiratory system and can be confused with the side effects of antipsychotic drugs.]

Benign Essential Blepharospasm Research Foundation
P.O. Box 12468
Beaumont, TX 77726
409-832-0788

▲ MENIERE'S DISEASE

[Meniere's disease is a poorly understood disease of unknown origin, character-ized by recurrent and severe dizziness, ringing in the ears (tinnitus), and possible hearing loss.]

American Tinnitus Association
P.O. Box 5
Portland, OR 97207
502-248-9985

The E.A.R. Foundation
ATTN.: Meniere's Network
2000 Church St.
Nashville, TN 37236
615-329-7807

The Vestibular Disorders Association
1015 22nd Ave., D-230
Portland, OR 97210-3079
503-229-7348

▲ MENTAL ILLNESS

National Alliance for the Mentally Ill
2101 Wilson Blvd.
Suite 302
Arlington, VA 22201
703-524-7600

▲ MIGRAINE

National Migraine Foundation
5252 North Western Ave.
Chicago, IL 60626
312-878-7715

▲ MULTIPLE SCLEROSIS

[Multiple sclerosis is a slowly progressive disease of the central nervous system with a great variety of symptoms, including abnormal sensations, weakness or clumsiness of limbs, visual disturbances, transient weakness, incontinence, and mild emotional disturbances. Because there is such a great variety of symptoms and no distinct biological marker, patients often must wait months or years for a diagnosis as doctors eliminate all other possibilities.]

National Multiple Sclerosis Society
202 East 42nd St.
New York, NY 10017
212-986-3240
800-624-8236 (hotline)

▲ MYALGIC ENCEPHALOMYELITIS

ME Association
P.O. Box 8
Stanford-le-Hope, Essex SS17 8EX
Great Britain

▲ MYASTHENIA GRAVIS

[Myasthenia gravis is a disease that involves fluctuating muscle weakness, with symptoms such as drooping eyelids, double vision, and muscle fatigue after exercise. Because of its rarity and rather vague symptoms, this disease is often misdiagnosed or dismissed.]

Myasthenia Gravis Foundation
53 West Jackson Blvd.
Suite 909
Chicago, IL 60604
312-427-6252
800-541-5454

▲ NARCOLEPSY

[Narcolepsy is a physical disorder characterized by recurrent attacks of sleep or drowsiness during the day, sudden loss of muscle tone (catalepsy), automatic behavior, sleep paralysis, and hallucinations just prior to sleep. Because there is no known biological marker and because all symptoms and signs are intense versions of normal behavior, narcolepsy is sometimes hard to distinguish from exhaustion, sleepiness, or neurotic fatigue.]

American Narcolepsy Association
P.O. Box 1187
San Carlos, CA 94070
415-591-7979

Narcolepsy and Cataplexy Foundation of America
Mail Box no. 22
1410 York Ave.
Suite 2D
New York, NY 10021
212-628-6315

▲ PAGET'S DISEASE
[Paget's disease is a metabolic disorder in which cells regulating bone tissue become overactive and produce excessive and abnormal new growth. It is often confused with arthritis or osteoporosis and with certain forms of cancer.]

Paget's Disease Foundation
P.O. Box 2772
Brooklyn, NY 11202
718-596-1043

▲ PARKINSON'S DISEASE
[Parkinson's disease is a slowly progressive, degenerative disease of the central nervous system, characterized by slowness of movement, muscular rigidity, tremor during rest, and unstable posture. It is often confused with essential tremor or various effects of aging.]

American Parkinson Disease Association
116 John St.
Suite 417
New York, NY 10038
212-732-9550
800-223-2732

Parkinson Support Groups of America
11376 Cherry Hill Rd., no. 204
Beltsville, MD 20705
301-937-1545

Parkinson's Educational Program—U.S.A.
1800 Park Newport, no. 302
Newport Beach, CA 92660
714-640-0218

United Parkinson Foundation
360 West Superior St.
Chicago, IL 60610
312-664-2344

▲ **PREMENSTRUAL SYNDROME**

PMS Access
P.O. Box 9326
Madison, WI 53715
608-833-4767

PMS Action
P.O. Box 16292
Irvine, CA 92713
(No phone number listed)

▲ **PUERPERAL MENTAL ILLNESS**

Depression after Delivery
P.O. Box 1282
Morrisville, PA 19067
215-295-3994

The Marcé Society
Institute of Psychiatry
De Crespigny Park
London SE5 8AF
England

▲ **RETT SYNDROME**

International Rett Syndrome Association
8511 Rose Marie Dr.
Fort Washington, MD 20744
301-248-7031

▲ REYE'S (REYE) SYNDROME

[Reye's or Reye syndrome is a children's disease that affects the liver and brain and has a mortality rate greater than 30 percent—death can occur within a few hours of onset. Cause and cure remain unknown, and questions about the relationship between aspirin and the syndrome remain. Reye's syndrome can be confused with poisoning or with encephalitis-like diseases.]

National Reye's Syndrome Foundation
426 North Lewis
Bryan, OH 43506
419-636-2679

▲ SCHIZOPHRENIA

American Schizophrenia Association
900 North Federal Highway, no. 330
Boca Raton, FL 33432
407-393-6167

▲ SJÖGREN'S SYNDROME

[Sjögren's syndrome is a common but often undiagnosed or misdiagnosed disorder marked by dry eyes, dry mouth, and often by connective-tissue disease such as rheumatoid arthritis or systemic lupus erythematosus.]

Sjögren's Syndrome Foundation
29 Gateway Dr.
Great Neck, NY 11021
516-487-2243
516-935-4380 (hotline)
718-347-1978 (hotline)
415-934-5826 (hotline)
616-496-7316 (hotline)

▲ SUDDEN INFANT DEATH SYNDROME

American Sudden Infant Death Syndrome Institute
800-232-SIDS (hotline)

National Center for the Prevention of Sudden Infant Death Syndrome (NCPSIDS)
330 North Charles St.
Baltimore, MD 21201
301-547-0300

National Sudden Infant Death Syndrome Clearinghouse
8201 Greensboro Dr.
Suite 600
McLean, VA 22102
703-821-8955

National Sudden Infant Death Syndrome Foundation
8200 Professional Pl.
Suite 104
Landover, MD 20795
301-459-3388
800-221-SIDS

Sudden Infant Death Syndrome Alliance
330 North Charles St.
Suite 203
Baltimore, MD 21201
301-837-8300
800-638-SIDS (hotline)

▲ TEMPEROMANDIBULAR JOINT SYNDROME

[TMJ syndrome is a painful disorder of the jaw joint; it worsens during or after eating or yawning. The jaw may have limited movement and may click and pop while chewing. Pain may also involve the eyes, ears, teeth, head, neck, shoulders, and back. Often difficult to diagnose, TMJ can be confused with rheumatoid arthritis, tinnitus, tetanus, migraine headache, sinus headache, earache, or chronic ear pain.]

Academy of Stress and Chronic Disease
1716 Hollingwood Dr.
Alexandria, VA 22307
(No phone number listed)

NIH/National Institute of Dental Research
9000 Rockville Pike
Bethesda, MD 20892
301-496-4261

The TMJ Education Association
840 Tanglewood Dr.
Brookfield, WI 53005
(No phone number listed)

▲ TOURETTE SYNDROME

Tourette Syndrome Association
42-40 Bell Blvd.
Bayside, NY 11361
718-224-2999
800-237-0717

▲ WILSON'S DISEASE

[Wilson's disease is a treatable and preventable (but often overlooked or mis-diagnosed) inherited disease in which the body cannot properly metabolize copper. Copper collects in various internal organs, leading both to physical signs and behavioral abnormalities. It is fatal if untreated.]

Wilson's Disease Association
P.O. Box 75324
Washington, DC 20013
703-636-3003

▲ GENERAL ORGANIZATIONS

▲ CHRONIC PAIN

American Chronic Pain Association
257 Old Haymaker Rd.
Monroeville, PA 15146
412-856-9676

National Chronic Pain Outreach Association
4922 Hampden La.
Bethesda, MD 20814
301-652-4948

▲ DEGENERATIVE DISEASES

National Organization for the Study of Degenerative Disease
P.O. Box 97
Ardsley, NY 10502
914-478-1862

▲ MISCELLANEOUS

American Self-Help Clearinghouse
St. Clare's-Riverside Medical Center
Pocono Rd.
Denville, NJ 07834
201-625-7101
[For $9.00 this group will send you the 3rd edition of *The Self-Help Sourcebook*, which contains information on more than 400 national self-help groups as well as numbers for more than 100 toll-free hotlines.]

Blackbag Bulletin Board List
29A-2 Golfview Dr.
Newark, DE 19702
(No phone number listed)
[This list, available for $5.00, is a guide to more than 300 computer-accessible health bulletin boards which can be particularly useful sources of self-help to the homebound.]

The Health Resource
209 Katherine Dr.
Conway, AR 72032
501-329-5272
[This medical research service provides individualized, in-depth research reports on specific health and medical problems, including little-understood or recognized diseases and hard-to-diagnose conditions. It also directs clients to support groups, reference materials, and alternative therapies.]

Long Distance Love
P.O. Box 2301
Ventnor, NJ 08406
(No phone number listed)
[This "pen pal" network uses a computerized file to put people with severe disabilities and chronic illnesses in touch with other people in similar circumstances.]

National Health Information Center
P.O. Box 1133
Washington, DC 20013-1133
800-336-4797
[This service supplies phone numbers for groups that help with specific diseases or medical problems, tapping into a computerized directory of more than 1,000 health-related organizations. For $1.00, the center will also provide a list of 125 health organizations that have toll-free telephone numbers.]

National Organization for Rare Disorders
P.O. Box 8923
New Fairfield, CT 06812
800-447-NORD

National Self-Help Clearinghouse
33 West 42nd St.
New York, NY 10036
212-642-2944

Notes

▲ INTRODUCTION. When Experts Disagree

1. See, for example, Edmond A. Murphy's discussion of diagnosis in his *Skepsis, Dogma, and Belief: Uses and Abuses in Medicine* (Baltimore: Johns Hopkins University Press, 1981), p. 142.

2. In at least a few published studies and in the introductions to the American Psychiatric Association's *Diagnostic and Statistical Manual of Mental Disorders* and its revision (DSM-III and DSM-III-R), academic psychiatrists recognize the need for common definitions of disease and disorder as well as the difficulty of finding them. For example, see Samuel B. Guze, "The Validity and Significance of the Clinical Diagnosis of Hysteria (Briquet's Syndrome)," *American Journal of Psychiatry* 1132 (1975): 138–141; id., "The Diagnosis of Hysteria: What Are We Trying to Do?" *American Journal of Psychiatry* 124 (1967): 491–498; id., "The Role of Follow-up Studies: Their Contribution to Diagnostic Classification as Applied to Hysteria," *Seminars in Psychiatry* 2 (1970): 392–402; and Robert L. Spitzer, Sally K. Severino, Janet B. W. Williams, and Barbara L. Parry, "Late Luteal Phase Dysphoric Disorder and DSM-III-R," *American Journal of Psychiatry* 146 (1989): 892–897. These works try to define mental disorder and disease in general, besides attempting to standardize definitions for specific disorders. How thoroughly these definitions are followed in the practical world of psychiatry, not to mention other medical specialties, however, remains debatable.

3. Susan Sontag, *Illness as Metaphor* (New York: Farrar, Straus & Giroux, 1977), p. 55.
4. *Dorland's Illustrated Medical Dictionary*, 25th ed. (Philadelphia: W. B. Saunders, 1974), s.v. "disease." "Etiology" refers to studying the factors that cause disease; "pathology" refers to studying the characteristics of disease; and "prognosis" refers to forecasting the probable outcome of a disease.
5. Ibid., s.v. "symptom."
6. Robert Hudson makes a similar point in his *Disease and Its Control* (New York: Praeger, 1987), p. 244.

▲ CHAPTER 1. Having an "In" Disease

1. *The Merck Manual of Diagnosis and Therapy*, 14th ed., ed. Robert Berkow (Rahway, N.J.: Merck, Sharp & Dohme Research Laboratories, 1982), s.v. "tetanus." Having a distinct etiology and/or therapy is by no means a necessary condition for an entity to be a disease, however. See Lester S. King, *Medical Thinking: A Historical Preface* (Princeton: Princeton University Press, 1982).
2. Linda Hanner emphasizes the importance of finding a diagnosis and details the frustrations of not finding one in her *When You're Sick and Don't Know Why: Coping with Your Undiagnosed Illness* (Minneapolis: DCI Publishing, 1991). Finding a name for a disease can also be comforting for the friends and family. As Sander Gilman shows in his *Disease and Representation: Images of Illness from Madness to AIDS* (Ithaca: Cornell University Press, 1988), assigning a specific and defined category to the sick person tends to distance the well from the suffering.
3. George Bernard Shaw, *Three Plays* (New York: New American Library, 1985), pp. 259, 312.
4. See, for example, George B. Markle IV, "Too Many of Us Are Just Plain Greedy," *Medical Economics*, February 6, 1989, pp. 23–30.
5. See, for example, Harry T. Paxton, "Why Doctors Get Sued," *Medical Economics*, April 18, 1988, pp. 42–50.
6. Robert A. Hamilton, "Rare Disease Treatments: 'Orphans' Saving Lives," *FDA Consumer* 24 (1990): 6–10.
7. For this information I am indebted to Irene Wielawska, who described Tammy's condition to me over the phone and reported it at length in two articles: "Daring to Hope, and Fight, to Find a Miracle for Tammy," *Providence Sunday Journal*, December 7, 1986; "The Fight for Tammy's 'Magic Cure.'" *Providence Journal*, December 8, 1986.
8. Bengt Hagberg, professor and chairman of pediatrics at the University of Gothenburg in Sweden, published his pathbreaking article on Rett syndrome in the October 1983 issue of the *Annals of Neurology*.

9. Ronald V. Norris, M.D., with Colleen Sullivan, *PMS: Premenstrual Syndrome* (New York: Berkley Books, 1984).

10. James Alexander Hamilton, "The Identity of Postpartum Psychosis," in *Motherhood and Mental Illness*, ed. I. F. Brockington and R. Kumar (New York: Grune & Stratton, 1982), pp. 1–17.

11. Terra Ziporyn, "'Rip Van Winkle Period' Ends for Puerperal Psychiatric Problems," *JAMA* 251 (1984): 2062.

12. See Terra Ziporyn, *Disease in the Popular American Press* (Westport, Conn.: Greenwood Press, 1988), and Susan Sontag, *Illness as Metaphor* (New York: Farrar, Straus & Giroux, 1977). For a brief overview of many of the ideas in this chapter, see Barbara Ehrenreich, "Sick Chic," *Ms.,* February 1989, pp. 28–29.

13. Graham Scrambler, "Perceiving and Coping with Stigmatizing Illness," in *The Experience of Illness*, ed. Ray Fitzpatrick et al. (New York: Tavistock Publications, 1984), pp. 212–213; Anthony Hopkins, *Epilepsy: The Facts* (Oxford: Oxford University Press, 1981), pp. 7, 52–53.

14. Even today, doctors believe that certain foods rich in chemicals called purines, from which the body makes uric acid, can exacerbate the disease—but they are not necessarily the cause of gout.

15. Frank E. James, "Office Pariahs: Sometimes the Stigma of Serious Illness Hurts More than the Disease Itself," *Wall Street Journal,* April 22, 1988.

16. Betty B. Osman, *Learning Disabilities: A Family Affair* (Mount Vernon, N.Y.: Consumers Union Edition, 1979), p. 27.

17. David Jobson, "Personal View," *British Medical Journal* 291 (1985): 599.

18. Julia Older, *Endometriosis* (New York: Charles Scribner's Sons, 1978), p. 144.

19. Ray Fitzpatrick, "Lay Concepts of Illness," in *The Experience of Illness,* p. 27. Knud Faber, in his early work on the meaning of diseases, noted that the practical value is obvious: "Nosography forms the basis of the whole of our diagnosis and of every form of treatment which is not purely symptomatic" (*Nosography: The Evolution of Clinical Medicine in Modern Times*, 2nd ed. [New York: Paul B. Hoeber, 1930; reprint, New York: AMS Press, 1978], p. viii).

20. Hopkins, *Epilepsy,* p. 85.

21. John Milne, "Sick Child Is Square Peg in System of Round Holes," *Boston Globe,* September 13, 1987. Eventually, Melanie received some funding because she was blind and fit that specific category for aid. In addition, a year later, partly through the efforts of Melanie's parents, New Hampshire passed legislation that allows some financial support for patients like Melanie who have undiagnosed diseases. As of late 1991, Melanie had not yet received a name for her condition, although magnetic-resonance imaging (MRI) has revealed a deterioration of the white matter of the brain. Melanie's mother, Tracy Broderick, says that the child's bodily functions continue to decline, to the point now that

she can no longer grasp objects and "her hips keep popping out." She describes her daughter's condition as "terminal."

22.   Bella English, "Living with Uncertainty," *Boston Globe,* March 11, 1987. Gregg Charles Fisher reports similar problems with obtaining Social Security benefits for chronic fatigue syndrome in the days when few physicians recognized that condition as a specific disease. See his *Chronic Fatigue Syndrome: A Victim's Guide to Understanding and Coping with This Debilitating Illness* (New York: Warner Books, 1989), pp. 110–129.

23.   "Epidemiologists to Consider Expanding AIDS Definition," *Boston Globe,* May 18, 1987. See also James and Kevin Helliker, "Alopecia Sufferers Seek to Suffer Less, and Not in Silence," *Wall Street Journal,* June 7, 1991. In August 1987, the Centers for Disease Control (CDC) revised their case definition to recognize only AIDS (generally defined as HIV infection together with one of many possible indicator diseases) as a statistical category. As of late 1991, the terms "AIDS," "ARC," and "HIV infection" continued to be used interchangeably in the lay press and even by some medical practitioners; but, according to a spokesman for the CDC, "We don't use the term 'ARC' as a category for gathering statistics. It means too many different things to different people." See Council of State and Territorial Epidemiologists, "Revision of the CDC Surveillance Case Definition for Acquired Immunodeficiency Syndrome," *MMWR* 36, supp. (1987): 3–15.

▲ CHAPTER 2. Having a "Nameless" Disease

1.   Unless otherwise indicated, all characters identified by first name are fictional composites based on the traits of many real patients. Characters denoted by initials or full names are actual patients, although I've changed a few details when necessary to protect their identities.

2.   I am using the word "condition" as a generic term that includes diseases, disorders, syndromes, and symptoms.

3.   Nameless diseases may include some of the "phantom" diseases described by Dr. Stuart Berger in his April 1987 *Good Housekeeping* article ("What to Do When Your Doctor Says There's Nothing Wrong with You and You Still Feel Awful"). According to Berger, phantom diseases "may come and go or the condition can appear to be another disease altogether" (p. 129).

4.   See, for example, Linda Hanner's *Lyme Disease: My Search for a Diagnosis* (Maple Plain, Minn.: Kashan Publishing, 1989).

5.   Susan Baur, *Hypochondria: Woeful Imaginations* (Berkeley: University of California Press, 1988), pp. 3–4. See also Phillip R. Slavney, *Perspectives on "Hysteria"* (Baltimore: Johns Hopkins University Press, 1990), pp. 34–55. According to Slavney (p. 2), the psychiatric community has

recently expunged the term "hysteria" from official diagnostic usage. The 3rd edition of their *Diagnostic and Statistical Manual of Mental Disorders* (DSM-III) renames "conversion hysteria" as "conversion disorder" and renames the personality type "hysterical" as "histrionic." Given the persistence of the terms "hysteria" and "hysterical" in both psychiatric literature and popular parlance, as well as the long history of the terms, however, I continue to use them here.

6. Terra Ziporyn, "'Rip Van Winkle Period' Ends for Puerperal Psychiatric Problems," *JAMA* 251 (1984): 2061–2067.

7. See, for example, Jane Dawson, "Royal Free Disease: Perplexity Continues," *British Medical Journal* 294 (1987): 327–328, and P. O. Behan and W. M. Behan, "Postviral Fatigue Syndrome," *Critical Review of Neurobiology* 4 (1988): 157–178.

8. John R. Paul, *A History of Poliomyelitis* (New Haven: Yale University Press, 1971), p. 200.

9. Ibid., p. 365.

10. See Lawrence K. Altman, "Syphilis Fools a New Generation," *New York Times,* November 13, 1990.

11. I. F. Brockington and R. Kumar, "Drug Addiction and Psychotropic Drug Treatment during Pregnancy and Lactation," in *Motherhood and Mental Illness,* ed. Brockington and Kumar (New York: Grune & Stratton, 1982), p. 239.

12. James Alexander Hamilton, "The Identity of Postpartum Psychosis," in *Motherhood and Mental Illness,* p. 11.

13. Remarkably, Hamilton reports, the woman "happily . . . survived all of this" and eventually became "productively employed in the electronics industry" (ibid., p. 12).

14. Ibid.

15. Anthony Hopkins, *Epilepsy: The Facts* (Oxford: Oxford University Press, 1981), p. 87.

16. For a more technical discussion of the importance of proper classification in research and census-taking, see Gerald N. Grob, *Edward Jarvis and the Medical World of Nineteenth-Century America* (Knoxville: University of Tennessee Press, 1978), p. 200.

17. See Larrian Gillespie, *You Don't Have to Live with Cystitis!* (New York: Rawson Associates, 1986).

18. *What Is Dyslexia?* (Baltimore: Orton Dyslexia Society, n.d.).

19. Speech by David M. Kaufman, M.D., at the 1985 annual meeting of the Orton Dyslexia Society, New York; Joel C. Don, "The Bright Ideas of Dyslexic Minds," *UCI Journal* (1986): 10–11.

20. Linda M. Watkins, "Premenstrual Distress Gains Notice as a Chronic Issue in the Workplace," *Wall Street Journal,* January 22, 1986.

21. A more narrow diagnosis, "late luteal phase dysphoric disorder," is instead included in a special appendix. See American Psychiatric Asso-

ciation, *Diagnostic and Statistical Manual of Mental Disorders,* rev. 3rd ed. (Washington, D.C.: American Psychiatric Association, 1987), pp. 367–369.

22.   Katharina Dalton, "Prophylactic Progesterone for Postnatal Depression" (MS, n.d.), p. 24.

23.   See H. Jane Chihal, *Premenstrual Syndrome: A Clinic Manual* (Durant, Okla.: Creative Infomatics, 1985), p. 9, and Elaine Blume, "Premenstrual Syndromes, Depression Linked," *JAMA* 249 (1983): 2864–2866.

24.   Carol Havens, "Premenstrual Syndrome: Tactics for Intervention," *Postgraduate Medicine* 77 (1985): 32–37.

25.   Ronald V. Norris, M.D., with Colleen Sullivan, *PMS: Premenstrual Syndrome* (New York: Berkley Books, 1984), pp. 12–15; Howard J. Osofsky, "Efficacious Treatments of PMS: A Need for Further Research," *JAMA* 264 (1990): 387.

26.   Uriel Halbreich, Jean Endicott, and John Nee, "Premenstrual Depressive Changes," *Archives of General Psychiatry* 40 (1983): 535–542; Joan Liebmann-Smith, "PMS, Insomnia . . . or Thyroid?" *American Health,* September 1985, pp. 76–81; Blume, "Premenstrual Syndromes."

27.   Ann L. Nazzaro and Donald R. Lombard, *The PMS Solution* (n.p.: Eden Press, 1985), p. 160.

28.   See, for example, R. E. Kendell, "The Concept of Disease and Its Implications for Psychiatry," *British Journal of Psychiatry* 127 (1975): 305–315; R. E. Kendell, *The Role of Diagnosis in Psychiatry* (Oxford: Blackwell, 1975); R. E. Kendell, J. E. Cooper, A. J. Gourlay, J.R.M. Copeland, L. Sharpe, and B. J. Gurland, "The Diagnostic Criteria of American and British Psychiatrists," *Archives of General Psychiatry* 25 (1971): 123–130; *Manual of the International Statistical Classification of Diseases, Injuries, and Causes of Death,* 9th ed. (Geneva: World Health Organization, 1977); J. D. Feighner et al., "Diagnostic Criteria for Use in Psychiatric Research," *Archives of General Psychiatry* 26 (1972): 57–63; E. Robins and S. B. Guze, "Classification of Affective Disorders: The Primary Secondary, the Endogenous Reactive, and the Neurotic-Psychotic Concepts," in *Recent Advances in the Psychobiology of the Depressive Illness,* ed. T. A. Williams, M. M. Katz, and J. A. Sheild (Washington, D.C.: U.S. Government Printing Office, 1972), pp. 283–293; E. Robins and S. B. Guze, "Establishment of Diagnostic Validity in Psychiatric Illness: Its Application to Schizophrenia," *American Journal of Psychiatry* 126 (1970): 107; Gerald L. Klerman, "Introduction," in *Treatment of Mental Disorders,* ed. John H. Greist, James W. Jefferson, and Robert L. Spitzer (New York: Oxford University Press, 1982), pp. xvii–xxviii; Robert L. Spitzer and Janet B. W. Williams, "Classification of Mental Disorders and DSM-III," in *Comprehensive Textbook of Psychiatry,* 3rd ed., ed. Harold I. Kaplan and Benjamin J. Sadock (Baltimore: Williams & Wilkins, 1981), pp. 1035–1056; K. Menninger, M. Mayman, and P. Pruyser, *The Vital*

Balance (New York: Viking, 1963); D. A. Rosenhan, "On Being Sane in Insane Places," *Science* 179 (1973): 250–258; and Thomas Szasz, *The Myth of Mental Illness* (New York: Harper & Row, 1974).

29.   James H. Cassedy, *American Medical and Statistical Thinking, 1800–1860* (Cambridge: Harvard University Press, 1984), pp. 157–168.

30.   Norris and Sullivan, *PMS*, p. 187.

31.   Some researchers do believe, however, that there may be some soft neurological signs. Children with dyslexia or with attention disorder syndrome may hold their hands in certain ways, grimace while walking, and so forth.

32.   Albert M. Galaburda et al., "Developmental Dyslexia: Four Consecutive Patients with Cortical Anomalies," *Annals of Neurology* 18 (1985): 222–233.

33.   Frank H. Duffy et al., "Dyslexia: Regional Differences in Brain Electrical Activity by Topographic Mapping," *Annals of Neurology* 7 (1980): 412–420.

34.   Gina Kolata, "New Clues to Complex Biology of Dyslexia," *New York Times*, December 8, 1987.

35.   Paul Raeburn, "Dyslexia Linked to Chromosome Defect," *Boston Globe*, November 5, 1986.

36.   Madeline Drexler, "Chronic Fatigue Syndrome," *Boston Globe Magazine*, November 4, 1990, pp. 46–47.

37.   A survey of 35 migrant and public health clinics in Texas, New Mexico, and Arizona included interviews with 1,341 people who identified themselves as "Mexican-American," 455 as "Mexican," 102 as "Spanish-American," and 2 as "Hispanic."

38.   R. T. Trotter, "Folk Medicine in the Southwest: Myths and Medical Facts," *Postgraduate Medicine* 78 (1985): 167–179. For another point of view, see Bernard Ortiz de Montellano's *Aztec Medicine, Health, and Nutrition* (New Brunswick: Rutgers University Press, 1990).

▲ CHAPTER 3. The Difficulty of Naming Diseases

1.   For more formal discussions of the process of diagnosis and its relationship to classification, see Lester S. King's "How Does a Pathologist Make a Diagnosis?" *Archives of Pathology* 84 (1967): 331–333, and his "The Meaning of Medical Diagnosis," *Etc.* 8 (1951): 202–211.

2.   The issue of what it means for something to "cause" a disease is another matter for complex philosophical debate and, in a more technical work, would deserve a chapter in its own right. For an excellent discussion of the complexities of the term "cause," see Lester S. King, *Medical Thinking: A Historical Preface* (Princeton: Princeton University Press, 1982), pp. 187–223. Here, however, I am using the noun "cause" as it is

commonly understood, to designate *any* of the factors we consider to be necessary (though not necessarily sufficient) prerequisites of the disease.

3. For philosophical discussions of the notion of disease, see Christopher Boorse, "Health as a Theoretical Concept," *Philosophy of Science* 44 (1977): 542–573; id., "On the Distinction between Disease and Illness," *Philosophy and Public Affairs* 5 (1975): 49–68; id., "What a Theory of Mental Health Should Be," *Journal for the Theory of Social Behaviour* 6 (1976): 61–84; L. J. Rather, "Towards a Philosophical Study of the Idea of Disease," in *The Historical Development of Physiological Thought,* ed. C. M. Brooks and P. F. Cranefield (New York: Hafner, 1959); J. G. Scadding, "Diagnosis: The Clinician and the Computer," *Lancet* 2 (1967): 877–882; E. J. M. Campbell, J. G. Scadding, and R. S. Roberts, "The Concept of Disease," *British Medical Journal* 2 (1979): 757–762; F. Kräupl Taylor, *The Concepts of Illness, Disease, and Morbus* (Cambridge: Cambridge University Press, 1979); Robert P. Hudson, *Disease and Its Control* (New York: Praeger, 1987); Robert P. Hudson, "The Concept of Disease," *Annals of Internal Medicine* 65 (1966): 595–601; Horacio Fabrega, Jr., "Concepts of Disease: Logical Features and Social Implications," *Perspectives in Biology and Medicine* 15 (1972): 583–616; Alvan R. Feinstein, "Clinical Epidemiology: I. The Populational Experiments of Nature and of Man in Human Illness," *Annals of Internal Medicine* 69 (1968): 807–820; Alvan R. Feinstein, "Clinical Epidemiology: II. The Identification Rates of Disease," *Annals of Internal Medicine* 69 (1968): 1037–1061; King, *Medical Thinking;* Lester S. King, "What Is Disease?" *Philosophy of Science* 21 (1954): 193–203; Arthur Kleinman, Leon Eisenberg, and Byron Good, "Culture, Illness, and Care: Clinical Lessons from Anthropologic and Cross-Cultural Research," *Annals of Internal Medicine* 88 (1978): 251–258; W. Riese, *The Conception of Disease* (New York: Philosophical Library, 1953); Arthur Kleinman, *The Illness Narratives: Suffering, Healing & the Human Condition* (New York: Basic Books, 1988); C. R. Burns, "Diseases versus Healths: Some Legacies in the Philosophies of Modern Medical Science," in *Evaluation and Explanation in the Biomedical Sciences,* ed. H. T. Engelhardt, Jr., and S. F. Spicker (Dordrecht: D. Reidel Publishing Co., 1975); H. Tristram Engelhardt, Jr., "The Concepts of Health and Disease," in *Evaluation and Explanation,* pp. 126–141; Susan Sontag, *Illness as Metaphor* (New York: Farrar, Straus & Giroux, 1977); *Concepts of Health and Disease,* ed. A. L. Caplan, H. T. Engelhardt, Jr., and J. J. McCartney (Reading, Mass.: Addison-Wesley, 1981); Laurence Foss and Kenneth Rothenberg, *The Second Medical Revolution: From Biomedicine to Infomedicine* (Boston: Shambhala, 1988); Richard H. Shryock, "The Interplay of Social and Internal Factors in the History of Modern Medicine," *Scientific Monthly* 76 (1953): 221–230; George L. Engel, "A Unified Concept of Health and Disease," *Perspectives in Biology and Medicine* 3 (1960): 459–485;

George L. Engel, "The Need for a New Medical Model: A Challenge for Biomedicine," *Science* 196 (1977): 129–136; and Owsei Temkin, "Health and Disease," in vol. 2 of the *Dictionary of the History of Ideas,* ed. Philip P. Wiener (New York: Charles Scribner's Sons, 1973), pp. 395–407.

4. Boorse, "Health as a Theoretical Concept," pp. 542–573. In fact, as Temkin observes, "Within this vast history [of ideas about health and disease], any order can be achieved only by neglecting innumerable details, by paradigmatic use of relatively few opinions and practices, and by admitting that a different point of view may show a different panorama" ("Health and Disease," p. 295).

5. One satisfactory definition, which encompasses every condition we might want to call "disease," comes from the medical philosopher Lester King: "Disease is the aggregate of those conditions which, judged by the prevailing culture, are deemed painful, or disabling, and which, at the same time, deviate from either the statistical norm or from some idealized status" ("What Is Disease?" p. 197).

6. Campbell, Scadding, and Roberts, "The Concept of Disease."

7. For a thorough philosophical discussion of questions like these, see King, *Medical Thinking,* pp. 169–175.

8. John C. Gunn, *Gunn's Domestic Medicine,* a facsimile of the 1st edition, with an introduction by Charles E. Rosenberg (Knoxville: University of Tennessee Press, Tennesseana Editions, 1986), pp. 149, 260–261. The book was originally published as *Gunn's Domestic Medicine; or, Poor Man's Friend* (Knoxville: "Printed under the immediate superintendence of the author, a physician of Knoxville," 1830).

9. Ibid., p. 203.

10. Feinstein, "Clinical Epidemiology: II," pp. 1038–1039. The attempt to derive a consistent classification of diseases and disorders in psychiatry began much later and, indeed, continues quite self-consciously to this day. As late as 1840 the U.S. census included only one category of mental illness—idiocy—and by 1880 the number of categories had only grown to seven: mania, melancholia, monomania, paresis, dementia, dipsomania, and epilepsy. Since 1889, psychiatrists, the World Health Organization, and various U.S. government agencies have attempted to design a standard nomenclature, originally attempting to classify mental conditions according to etiology and later relying on more descriptive criteria.

During the past two decades, further revisions have been made, based on significant methodological developments in the study of the diagnostic process, new diagnostic techniques, and new ways to classify and define the diagnostic categories: cross-national studies, computer programs, mathematically derived diagnostic types, specific diagnostic criteria, structured interviews, epidemiological community surveys, and multiaxial classification (which helps differentiate people who share a single symptom but who otherwise have different characteristics). The culmination of these efforts is the revised third edition of the American Psychiatric Association's *Diagnostic and Statistical Manual of Mental Disorders.* For details, see Robert L. Spitzer and Janet B. W. Williams, "Classification of Mental Disorders and DSM-III," in *Comprehensive Textbook of Psychiatry,* 3rd ed., ed. Harold I. Kaplan and Benjamin J. Sadock (Baltimore: Williams & Wilkins, 1981), pp. 1044–1052, and Gerald L. Klerman, "Introduction," in *Treatment of Mental Disorders,* ed. John H. Greist, James W. Jefferson, and Robert L. Spitzer (New York: Oxford University Press, 1982), pp. xvii–xxviii.

11. Taylor, *The Concepts of Illness,* pp. 6–11; Knud Faber, *Nosography: The Evolution of Clinical Medicine in Modern Times,* 2nd ed. (New York: Paul B. Hoeber, 1930; reprint, New York: AMS Press, 1978), pp. 8–9.

12. Faber, *Nosography,* pp. 11–12.

13. Ibid., pp. 20–21; Hudson, *Disease and Its Control,* pp. 236–237.

14. Lester S. King, *The Medical World of the Eighteenth Century* (Chicago: University of Chicago Press, 1958), pp. 198–199.

15. Taylor calls this clincher the "radical source indicator." See his chapter "Source Indicators and Their Perception," in *The Concepts of Illness,* pp. 32–45.

16. Ibid., pp. 199–200, 209–210, 214–218; James H. Cassedy, *American Medical and Statistical Thinking, 1800–1860* (Cambridge: Harvard University Press, 1984), pp. 22–23.

17. King, *The Medical World of the Eighteenth Century,* pp. 220, 222–223.

18. Many people today are again beginning to verify the validity of psychically induced symptoms, but the notion is not generally recognized in the medical literature.

19. See Hudson's chapter "Disease as Localized," in his *Disease and Its Control,* pp. 101–119, and Faber, *Nosography,* p. 37.

20. Faver, *Nosography,* pp. 28–30.

21. This was originally pointed out by Dr. William Farr (1839–1880), superintendent with the statistical department of Britain's General Register Office. See Gerald N. Grob, *Edward Jarvis and the Medical World of Nineteenth-Century America* (Knoxville: University of Tennessee Press, 1978), p. 93.

22. *Manual of the International Statistical Classification of Diseases, Injuries, and Causes of Death* (Geneva: World Health Organization, 1967), p. vii.

23. Grob, *Edward Jarvis,* p. 92.

24. See Taylor, *The Concepts of Illness,* pp. 93–94.

25. Faber, *Nosography,* pp. 116–125; see also Feinstein, "Clinical Epidemiology: II, pp. 1038–1039.

26. Faber, *Nosography,* pp. 150–151.

27. Ibid., p. 177.

28. King, *Medical Thinking,* pp. 158–159.

29.   Ibid., pp. 66–67.

30.   Ibid., p. 68.

31.   Note that by listing the objects in this way, I have already classified them, if unconsciously.

32.   For a discussion of the difficulty of arranging empirically observed entities (such as patients) exactly, see Taylor's chapter "Classes and Classifications," in *The Concepts of Disease,* pp. 46–59.

▲ **CHAPTER 4.** Are There Really Any Diseases?

1.   Harold Bursztajn et al., *Medical Choices, Medical Chances: How Patients, Families, and Physicians Can Cope with Uncertainty* (New York: Delacorte Press/Seymour Lawrence, 1981), pp. 3–19.

2.   See, for example, Robert P. Hudson's chapter "Health, Disease, and Illness," in his *Disease and Its Control* (New York: Praeger, 1987), pp. 229–247.

3.   Georges Canguilhem, *On the Normal and the Pathological,* trans. Carolyn R. Fawcett (Dordrecht: D. Reidel Publishing Co., 1978), p. 12; Hudson, *Disease and Its Control,* pp. 84–85, 234; H. Tristram Engelhardt, Jr., "The Concepts of Health and Disease," in *Evaluation and Explanation in the Biomedical Sciences,* ed. H. T. Engelhardt, Jr., and S. F. Spicker (Dordrecht: D. Reidel Publishing Co., 1975), pp. 126–141.

4.   Lester S. King, *Medical Thinking: A Historical Preface* (Princeton: Princeton University Press, 1982), pp. 132–135.

5.   Rush's system was based on that of the British physician John Brown. See Benjamin Rush, "Outlines of the Phenomena of Fever," in *Medical Inquiries and Observations* (Philadelphia: Johnson & Warner et al., 1809), vol. 3, pp. 7–17, 33–34; James H. Cassedy, *American Medical and Statistical Thinking, 1800–1860* (Cambridge: Harvard University Press, 1984), pp. 21, 53ff.; Richard H. Shryock, "Benjamin Rush from the Perspective of the Twentieth Century," in *Medicine in America: Historical Essays,* ed. Richard H. Shryock (Baltimore: Johns Hopkins University Press, 1966), pp. 233–251; Lester S. King, *The Medical World of the Eighteenth Century* (Chicago: University of Chicago Press, 1958), p. 223; John Harley Warner, *The Therapeutic Perspective: Medical Practice, Knowledge, and Identity in America, 1820–1885* (Cambridge: Harvard University Press, 1986); and Hudson, *Disease and Its Control,* p. 238.

6.   King, *Medical Thinking,* pp. 135–137.

7.   Lynn Payer, *Medicine & Culture* (New York: Henry Holt & Co., 1988), pp. 61–67, 73, 92.

8.   David Eisenberg, M.D., with Thomas Lee Wright, *Encounters with Qi: Exploring Chinese Medicine* (New York: W. W. Norton, 1985), pp. 55–59.

9. For example, see F. Kräupl Taylor, *The Concepts of Illness, Disease, and Morbus* (Cambridge: Cambridge University Press, 1979), pp. 17–31.

10. Arthur Kleinman, *The Illness Narratives: Suffering, Healing & the Human Condition* (New York: Basic Books, 1988), pp. 228–229.

11. See Hudson, *Disease and Its Control*, pp. 87, 98–99, 102; Warner, *The Therapeutic Perspective*, pp. 87, 235–257; and Knud Faber, *Nosography: The Evolution of Clinical Medicine in Modern Times*, 2nd ed. (New York: Paul B. Hoeber, 1930; reprint, New York: AMS Press, 1978), pp. vi–vii.

12. King, *The Medical World of the Eighteenth Century*, p. 196. For similar arguments see Faber, *Nosography*, p. 186; Edmond A. Murphy, "The Ontology of Nonexistents," in Murphy's *Skepsis, Dogma, and Belief: Uses and Abuses in Medicine* (Baltimore: Johns Hopkins University Press, 1981), pp. 43–60; and Gerald N. Grob, *Edward Jarvis and the Medical World of Nineteenth-Century America* (Knoxville: University of Tennessee Press, 1978), pp. 68–69.

13. King, *Medical Thinking*, p. 110; Faber, *Nosography*, p. 27; Grob, *Edward Jarvis*, pp. 68–69.

14. For more detailed discussion of the historical development of psychiatric nomenclature and nosology, see Gerald L. Klerman, "Introduction," in *Treatment of Mental Disorders*, ed. John H. Greist, James W. Jefferson, and Robert L. Spitzer (New York: Oxford University Press, 1982), pp. xvii–xxviii, and Robert L. Spitzer and Janet B. W. Williams, "Classification of Mental Disorders and DSM-III," in *Comprehensive Textbook of Psychiatry*, 3rd ed. (Baltimore: Williams & Wilkins, 1981), pp. 1035–1056.

15. Emil Kraepelin, "Manic-Depressive Insanity and Paranoia," trans. R. Mary Barclay, in *Textbook of Psychiatry*, 8th ed., ed. George M. Robertson (Edinburgh: E.B.S. Livingston, 1921), p. 2.

16. Psychiatrists still distinguish between diseases and disorders: diseases represent a disturbed anatomical structure, while disorders represent a disturbed physiological function. Presumably, improved technology will blur the boundaries between these two categories. See Taylor, *The Concepts of Illness*, p. 94.

17. King, *Medical Thinking*, pp. 123–124, 126–127.

18. For an excellent discussion of the use and abuse of reification, see Stephen Jay Gould's *The Mismeasure of Man* (New York: W. W. Norton, 1981), p. 24 et passim.

19. Terra Ziporyn, "'Rip Van Winkle Period' Ends for Puerperal Psychiatric Problems," *JAMA* 251 (1984): 2061.

20. Taylor makes a similar point (*The Concepts of Illness*, p. 6) as does George L. Engel in "A Unified Concept of Health and Disease," *Perspectives in Biology and Medicine* 3 (1960): 460.

21. Faber, *Nosography*, pp. 47–48. See also Hudson, *Disease and Its Con-*

trol, pp. 239–240, and Warner, *The Therapeutic Perspective,* pp. 48–49.

22. Faber, *Nosography,* pp. 48–49.
23. Ibid., pp. 66–67, 70, 77–79. See also Warner, *The Therapeutic Perspective,* pp. 281–282, and Taylor, who shows that the older Virchow adopted an ontological outlook (*The Concepts of Illness,* pp. 11–16, 17–20, 74, 76).
24. Charles E. Rosenberg, "Introduction to the New Edition," in John C. Gunn, *Gunn's Domestic Medicine* (Knoxville: University of Tennessee Press, Tennesseana Editions, 1986), p. xii. This book was originally published as *Gunn's Domestic Medicine; or, Poor Man's Friend* (Knoxville: "Printed under the immediate superintendence of the author, a physician of Knoxville," 1830).
25. Rush, "Outlines," p. 34.
26. Warner, *The Therapeutic Perspective,* pp. 58–80; Charles Rosenberg, "The Therapeutic Revolution: Medicine, Meaning, and Social Change in Nineteenth-Century America," in *The Therapeutic Revolution: Essays in the Social History of American Medicine,* ed. Morris J. Vogel and Charles E. Rosenberg (Philadelphia: University of Pennsylvania Press, 1979).
27. Rush, "Outlines," p. 35.
28. Gunn, *Gunn's Domestic Medicine,* p. 129.
29. Warner, *The Therapeutic Perspective,* p. 18; Faber, *Nosography,* p. 110.
30. Erwin H. Ackerknecht, *Medicine at the Paris Hospital: 1794–1848* (Baltimore: Johns Hopkins University Press, 1967), pp. 68–70.
31. As Warner argues quite persuasively in *The Therapeutic Perspective,* this trend was ending even before bacteriology had shown any concrete therapeutic results. The reasons were numerous, including professional pressures, an increasing reliance on instrumentation, and an emphasis on scientific medicine (pp. 37–57).
32. Faber, *Nosography,* pp. 207–208.
33. Louis Goldman, "Premenstrual Syndrome: Is It Oversold or Underdiagnosed?" *Modern Medicine,* June 1985, p. 16. See also Anthony Hopkins, *Epilepsy: The Facts* (Oxford: Oxford University Press, 1981), p. 7, who explains that the decision of when to diagnose epilepsy is based on convenience.
34. Edmund D. Pellegrino, "Essay: The Sociocultural Impact of Twentieth-Century Therapeutics," in *The Therapeutic Revolution: Essays in the Social History of American Medicine,* ed. Morris J. Vogel and Charles E. Rosenberg (Philadelphia: University of Pennsylvania Press, 1979), pp. 245–266.
35. For examples of alternative ways to group phenomena into a disease category, see Bursztajn et al., *Medical Choices;* George L. Engel, "The Need for a New Medical Model: A Challenge for Biomedicine," *Science* 196 (1977): 129–136; Laurence Foss and Kenneth Rothenberg, *The Sec-*

ond Medical Revolution: From Biomedicine to Infomedicine (Boston: New Science Library, 1988); and Kleinman, *The Illness Narratives.*

36.   Hudson, *Disease and Its Control,* p. 230.
37.   See Engel, "The Need for a New Medical Model," p. 463, and Lester S. King, "The Meaning of Medical Diagnosis," *Etc.* 8 (1951): 202–211.
38.   See, for example, Lester S. King, "What Is Disease?" *Philosophy of Science* 21 (1954): 193–203.

▲ CHAPTER 5. Mistaking Symptoms for Diseases

1.   David Steinberg, *Anemia* (Philadelphia: W. B. Saunders, 1982), p. 3.
2.   Ibid., pp. 1–2. For an analogous discussion of hypoglycemia, see Lynn J. Bennon, *Hypoglycemia, Fact or Fad? What You Should Know about Low Blood Sugar* (Mount Vernon, N.Y.: Consumers Union, 1986), p. 91.
3.   Steinberg, *Anemia,* p. 1.
4.   Bennon, *Hypoglycemia,* pp. 1–2.
5.   Ibid., p. 6.
6.   Ibid., pp. 3–4.
7.   Anthony Hopkins, *Epilepsy: The Facts* (Oxford: Oxford University Press, 1981), pp. 7–8. See also F. Kräupl Taylor, *The Concepts of Illness, Disease, and Morbus* (Cambridge: Cambridge University Press, 1979), pp. 32–45.
8.   "Chronic Migraines Hit Young People Hard," *Wall Street Journal,* June 7, 1991. Oliver Sacks, in *Migraine: Understanding a Common Disorder* (Berkeley: University of California Press, 1986), demonstrates that people who suffer from migraines represent a diverse, heterogeneous group and that migrainous conditions themselves, although they share certain characteristics, probably represent a heterogeneous group of related conditions with various etiologies. "There is probably no field in medicine," he observes, "so strewn with the debris of misdiagnosis and mistreatment, and of well-intentioned but wholly mistaken medical and surgical interventions" (p. 52).
9.   Ronald V. Norris, M.D., with Colleen Sullivan, *PMS: Premenstrual Syndrome* (New York: Berkley Books, 1984).
10.   Ann L. Nazzaro and Donald R. Lombard, *The PMS Solution* (n.p.: Eden Press, 1985).
11.   Ibid., p. ii.
12.   The researcher himself acknowledges that not all women with PMS have elevated prolactin levels, so this cannot be the sole cause.
13.   Carol Dix, *The New Mother Syndrome* (Garden City, N.Y.: Doubleday, 1985), pp. 108–122. Chapters trace postpartum depression to social factors such as the role of women in today's society, marital stresses, or difficult family situations, implying that PPD has less to do with hormones than with emotions.

14. Jesse A. Stoff and Charles R. Pellegrino, *Chronic Fatigue Syndrome: The Hidden Epidemic* (New York: Random House, 1988). The book is also repetitious, full of factual errors, and displays a misleading veneer of valid scientific thinking. See also Jane Meredith Adams, "Baffling Illness Yields New Clues: But No Cure in Sight for Chronic Fatigue," *Boston Globe*, May 29, 1989.

15. Betty B. Osman, *Learning Disabilities: A Family Affair* (Mount Vernon, N.Y.: Consumers Union, 1979), p. 4.

16. I recently heard an amazing statistic from some acquaintances in the education field: as many as 40 percent of all public school children are now classified as "learning disabled."

17. *Dorland's Illustrated Medical Dictionary*, 25th ed. (Philadelphia: W. B. Saunders, 1974), s.v. "symptom." See also Lester S. King's *Medical Thinking: A Historical Preface* (Princeton: Princeton University Press, 1982), p. 81, and his *Transformations in American Medicine: From Benjamin Rush to William Osler* (Baltimore: Johns Hopkins University Press, 1990), pp. 29–30.

18. The dizziness, headache, fatigue, nervousness, and other "symptoms" that may be experienced by people with hypertension arise from complications of hypertension in certain organs; they do not characterize the condition itself.

19. *Medical World News*, March 19, 1986, p. 100.

20. Benjamin Rush, "Outlines of the Phenomena of Fever," in *Medical Inquiries and Observations*, 3rd ed. (Philadelphia: Johnson & Warner et al., 1809), vol. 2, pp. 226–255, and vol. 3, pp. 3–66, 385–393; Lester S. King, "The Medical Milieu of Daniel Drake," *JAMA* 253 (1985): 2127; and King, *Transformations*, p. 43.

21. William Buchan, *Domestic Medicine* (New York: Garland Publishing, 1985), pp. 194–195.

22. John C. Gunn, *Gunn's Domestic Medicine*, a facsimile of the 1st edition, with an introduction by Charles E. Rosenberg (Knoxville: University of Tennessee Press, Tennesseana Editions, 1986), pp. 149, 199; the book was originally published as *Gunn's Domestic Medicine; or, Poor Man's Friend* (Knoxville: "Printed under the immediate superintendence of the author, a physician of Knoxville," 1830).

23. Lester S. King, *The Medical World of the Eighteenth Century* (Chicago: University of Chicago Press, 1958), p. 201. Also see Knud Faber, *Nosography: The Evolution of Clinical Medicine in Modern Times*, 2nd ed. (New York: Paul B. Hoeber, 1930; reprint, New York: AMS Press, 1978), p. 26.

24. Gunn, *Gunn's Domestic Medicine*, pp. 133–136.

25. Ibid., p. 140.

26. King, *Transformations*, pp. 138–141.

27. King, *The Medical World*, p. 202.

▲ **CHAPTER 6.** Mistaking Syndromes for Diseases

1.   Lester S. King, *Medical Thinking: A Historical Preface* (Princeton: Princeton University Press, 1982), p. 162; conversation with Dr. Marvin Lipman, Consumers Union medical adviser; *Understanding AIDS: A Comprehensive Guide,* ed. Victor Gong (New Brunswick: Rutgers University Press, 1985), pp. 1, 30.

2.   See, for example, Julia Older, *Endometriosis* (New York: Charles Scribner's Sons, 1978), pp. 18–19; Ronald V. Norris, M.D., with Colleen Sullivan, *PMS: Premenstrual Syndrome* (New York: Berkley Books, 1984), passim; and *Understanding AIDS,* passim.

3.   "Chronic Fatigue Syndrome," *Harvard Medical School Health Letter* 13 (1988): 1–3. See also G. P. Holmes et al., "Chronic Fatigue Syndrome: A Working Case Definition," *Annals of Internal Medicine* 108 (1988): 387–389; G. P. Holmes et al., "A Cluster of Patients with a Chronic Mononucleosis-like Syndrome: Is Epstein-Barr Virus the Cause?" *JAMA* 257 (1987): 2297–2302.

4.   Richard A. Knox, "The Baffling 'Chronic Mono' Syndrome," *Boston Globe,* January 12, 1987. Also see Knox's "Study Calls Fatigue Illness Widespread," *Boston Globe,* May 1, 1987.

5.   According to the psychiatrist Marvin C. Ziporyn, today most psychiatrists prefer to call this condition "bipolar disorder," although the name "manic-depressive disorder" is still common in lay circles.

6.   James B. Wyngaarden, "Disorders of Purine and Pyrimidine Metabolism: Gout," in *Cecil Textbook of Medicine,* 16th ed., ed. James B. Wyngaarden and Lloyd H. Smith (Philadelphia: W. B. Saunders, 1982), vol. 1, pp. 1107–1108.

7.   Norris and Sullivan, *PMS.* See also "The Case for PMS as a Legal Defense," *PMS Access,* May–June 1986, pp. 2–3.

8.   Except in the appendix to the American Psychiatric Association's DMS-III-R, which has more specific criteria for the related or perhaps identical mental condition currently called "late luteal phase dysphoric disorder." See Introduction, n. 2, above, and Robert L. Spitzer, Sally K. Severino, Janet B. W. Williams, and Barbara L. Parry, "Late Luteal Phase Dysphoric Disorder and DSM-III-R," *American Journal of Psychiatry* 146 (1989): 892–897.

9.   Conversations with William R. Keye, M.D., associate professor of obstetrics and gynecology at the University of Utah, Salt Lake City; with a clinician from the PMS Clinic at Duke University Medical Center, Durham, N.C.; and with Dr. Maureen Dalton, who studies PMS in Leeds, England. See also H. Jane Chihal, *Premenstrual Syndrome: A Clinic Manual* (Durant, Okla.: Creative Infomatics, 1985), pp. 39, 9–19, 103, and David Rubinow et al., "Menstrually Related Mood Disorders: Methodological and Conceptual Issues," in *Premenstrual Syndrome and Dys-*

menorrhea, ed. M. Yusoff Dawood, John L. McGuire, and Laurence Demers (Baltimore: Urban & Schwartzenberg, 1985).

10. See, for example, G. Stein, "The Maternity Blues," in *Motherhood and Mental Illness,* ed. I. F. Brockington and R. Kumar (New York: Grune & Stratton, 1982), pp. 136–137.

11. For an example of the kind of skepticism that this kind of liberal naming evokes and a discussion of the desire to connect vague psychological states with organic diseases, see Caroline Richmond, "Myalgic Encephalomyelitis, Princess Aurora, and the Wandering Womb," *British Medical Journal* 298 (1989): 1295–1296.

12. Francine Klagsbrun, "Debunking the 'Adopted Child Syndrome,'" *Ms.,* October 1986, p. 102.

13. *The Merck Manual of Diagnosis and Therapy,* 14th ed., ed. Robert Berkow (Rahway, N.J.: Merck, Sharp & Dohme Research Laboratories, 1982), pp. 1855–1856; Daniel Q. Haney, "MGH Study Links Crib Death, Heart Defects," *Boston Globe,* December 10, 1987.

14. As of July 18, 1987, the woman had been found guilty of smothering one infant daughter, and the county prosecutor had announced plans to prosecute her on charges of killing at least two of her other eight children. See Joe Mahoney, "N.Y. Mother Found Guilty of Smothering Infant Daughter," *Boston Globe,* July 18, 1987. Final verdict: guilty.

15. See Anthony Hopkins, *Epilepsy: The Facts* (Oxford: Oxford University Press, 1981), pp. 22–23.

16. *Cecil Textbook of Medicine,* vol. 2, p. 2114.

17. Betty B. Osman, *Learning Disabilities: A Family Affair* (Mount Vernon, N.Y.: Consumers Union, 1979), pp. 5, 6 (note), 20–21.

18. Ann L. Nazzaro and Donald R. Lombard, *The PMS Solution* (n.p.: Eden Press, 1985), pp. 5–6.

▲ **CHAPTER 7.** How Diseases Come and Go

1. For another conceptualization of this phenomenon, see Robert P. Hudson's chapter "The Birth and Death of Diseases," in his *Disease and Its Control* (New York: Praeger, 1987), pp. 3–20.

2. Knud Faber, *Nosography: The Evolution of Clinical Medicine in Modern Times,* 2nd ed. (New York: Paul B. Hoeber, 1930; reprint, New York: AMS Press, 1978), pp. 19–20.

3. Ibid., p. 39. See also Erwin H. Ackerknecht, *Medicine at the Paris Hospital: 1794–1848* (Baltimore: Johns Hopkins University Press, 1967), and Esmond R. Long, *A History of Pathology* (New York: Dover Publications, 1967).

4. David Steinberg, *Anemia* (Philadelphia: W. B. Saunders, 1982), pp. 67–72.

5.   Faber, *Nosography*, p. 37.

6.   Julia Older, *Endometriosis* (New York: Charles Scribner's Sons, 1978), p. 181.

7.   Ibid., p. 5.

8.   Ibid., p. 171.

9.   John C. Gunn, *Gunn's Domestic Medicine*, a facsimile of the 1st edition, with an introduction by Charles E. Rosenberg (Knoxville: University of Tennessee Press, Tennesseana Editions, 1986), pp. 303–305; originally *Gunn's Domestic Medicine; or, Poor Man's Friend* (Knoxville: "Printed under the immediate superintendence of the author, a physician of Knoxville," 1830). Also see R. V. Pierce, *The People's Common Sense Medical Adviser*, 8th ed. (Buffalo: World's Dispensary Printing-Office and Bindery, 1880), pp. 732–737, and R. V. Pierce, *The People's Common Sense Medical Adviser* (Buffalo: World's Dispensary Printing-Office and Bindery, 1895), pp. 702–706.

10.   See Harry F. Dowling, *Fighting Infection: Conquests of the Twentieth Century* (Cambridge: Harvard University Press, 1977), pp. 56–57, for more details. In her "Puerperal Fever in Eighteenth-Century Britain," *Bulletin of the History of Medicine* 63 (1989): 521–556, Margaret De-Lacy questions the view that puerperal fever was spread by germs left on hands after autopsies, suggesting instead that most cases were spread by doctors who were disease carriers during various epidemics.

11.   Gunn, *Gunn's Domestic Medicine*, p. 88.

12.   For example, recent research indicates that people with alcoholism may have livers that metabolize alcohol differently than those of non-alcoholics and that their central nervous systems may have lower levels of the enzyme monoamine oxidase. See Nicholas A. Pace's letter in the *New York Times* for November 27, 1987.

13.   "Phototherapy, Sleep Deprivation Effective Nondrug Treatments," *Psychiatric News*, November 21, 1986, p. 15. See also Peg Boyles, "New Light on Winter Darkness," *Yankee*, February 1988, pp. 107–111, 152–155.

14.   Arthur Kleinman, *The Illness Narratives: Suffering, Healing, and the Human Condition* (New York: Basic Books, 1989), p. 109.

15.   The American Psychiatric Association also decided to call this condition "late luteal phase dysphoric disorder," recognizing the fact that some nonmenstruating women with intact ovaries experience "PMS" and emphasizing the mood changes—not purely physical symptoms—necessary for its inclusion in a psychiatric manual. See Robert L. Spitzer, Sally K. Severino, Janet B. W. Williams, and Barbara L. Parry, "Late Luteal Phase Dysphoric Disorder and DSM-III-R," *American Journal of Psychiatry* 146 (1989): 892–897, and *New York Times*, July 6, 1986.

16.   Dora B. and Herbert Weiner, "Histoire de l'hystérie," *Bulletin of the History of Medicine* 61 (1987): 471–472. Also see Owsei Temkin, *The Fall-*

ing Sickness, 2nd ed. (Baltimore: Johns Hopkins University Press, 1971); Ilza Veith, *Hysteria, the History of a Disease* (Chicago: University of Chicago Press, 1965); and Phillip R. Slavney, *Perspectives on "Hysteria"* (Baltimore: Johns Hopkins University Press, 1990).

17.   See Guenter B. Risse's review of Georges Didi-Huberman, *Invention de l'hystérie. Charcot et l'iconographie photographique de la Salpêtrière* (Paris: Editions Macula, 1982), in the *Bulletin of the History of Medicine* 60 (1986): 269–270. "Prolapsed mitral valve syndrome" (PMVS), briefly recognized as a legitimate disease in the late 1970s, is another example of a short-lived disease (although many people still have to live with the same symptoms, with or without official recognition). See Barbara Ehrenreich, "Sick Chic," *Ms.,* February 1989, pp. 28–29.

18.   Barry Werth, "How Short Is Too Short," *New York Times Magazine,* June 14, 1991, pp. 14–17, 28–29, 47.

19.   Again, as pointed out above in Chapter 5, some conditions labeled as "syndromes" are actually diseases for all intents and purposes.

20.   Terra Ziporyn, "'Rip Van Winkle Period' Ends for Puerperal Psychiatric Problems," *JAMA* 251 (1984): 2061–2067.

21.   Oliver Sacks, too, in his book *The Man Who Mistook His Wife for a Hat* (New York: Summit Books, 1985), has a chapter ("Witty Ticcy Ray") about a man with Tourette syndrome.

22.   I. F. Brockington, G. Winokur, and Christine Dean, "Puerperal Psychosis," in *Motherhood and Mental Illness,* ed. I. F. Brockington and R. Kumar (New York: Grune & Stratton, 1982), p. 40.

23.   Ibid., p. 42.

24.   James Alexander Hamilton, "The Identity of Postpartum Psychosis," in *Motherhood and Mental Illness,* pp. 1–2.

25.   Ibid., p. 14.

26.   Ibid.

27.   Ziporyn, "'Rip Van Winkle Period' Ends," p. 2061.

28.   Katharina Dalton, "Prophylactic Progesterone for Postnatal Depression" (MS, n.d.), p. 156. To my knowledge, there is no conclusive study linking premenstrual syndrome and puerperal mental illness, although I've heard anecdotal accounts from researchers.

29.   Sacks, *The Man Who Mistook His Wife,* p. 90.

30.   Hudson, *Disease and Its Control,* pp. 6, 9.

31.   M. A. Crowther, "'Savill's Disease': A Pauper Epidemic in Britain and Its Implications," *Bulletin of the History of Medicine* 60 (1986): 556.

32.   See Marsha F. Goldsmith, "Not There Yet, but 'on Our Way' in AIDS Research, Scientists Say," *JAMA* 2543 (1985): 3369; Richard M. Selik, Harry W. Haverkos, and James W. Curran, "Acquired Immunodeficiency Syndrome (AIDS) Trends in the United States, 1978–1982," *American Journal of Medicine* 76 (1984): 493; Michael S. Gottlieb et al., "*Pneumocystis carinii* Pneumonia and Mucosal Candidiasis in Previously

Healthy Homosexual Men: Evidence of a New Acquired Cellular Immunodeficiency," *New England Journal of Medicine* 305 (1981): 1428; A. S. Fauci et al., "Acquired Immunodeficiency Syndrome: Epidemiologic, Clinical, Immunologic, and Therapeutic Considerations," *Annals of Internal Medicine* 100 (1984): 92; Henry Masur et al., "An Outbreak of Community-Acquired *Pneumocystis carinii* Pneumonia," *New England Journal of Medicine* 305 (1981): 1431–1438; and *Understanding AIDS: A Comprehensive Guide,* ed. Victor Gong (New Brunswick: Rutgers University Press, 1985), pp. 10–11.

33. Masur et al., "An Outbreak," p. 1431.

34. Gottlieb et al., "*Pneumocystis carinii* Pneumonia," pp. 1429–1430; Masur et al., "An Outbreak," p. 1436.

35. J. M. Guerin et al., "Widening the Definition of AIDS" (letter), *Lancet* 1 (1984): 1464–1465.

36. Fauci et al., "Acquired Immunodeficiency Syndrome," p. 92; *Understanding AIDS,* p. xi.

37. Fauci et al., "Acquired Immunodeficiency Syndrome," p. 92.

38. Margaret M. Heckler, "The Challenge of Acquired Immunodeficiency Syndrome," *Annals of Internal Medicine* 103 (1985): 655.

39. Paul A. Volberding, "The Clinical Spectrum of the Acquired Immunodeficiency Syndrome: Implications for Comprehensive Patient Care," *Annals of Internal Medicine* 103 (1985): 730–731; Michael Marsh, Victor Gong, and Daniel Shindler, "Questions and Answers about AIDS," in *Understanding AIDS,* p. 191.

40. Charles Marwick, "'Molecular Level' View Gives Immune System Clues," *JAMA* 253 (1985): 3371.

41. John T. MacFarlane, "Legionnaire's Disease," *Practitioner* 227 (1983): 1707–1718. See also volume 90 of the *Annals of Internal Medicine* (1979) in its entirety.

42. MacFarlane, "Legionnaire's Disease," p. 1709.

43. *Understanding AIDS,* p. 77.

44. J. B. Brunet and R. A. Ancelle, "The International Occurrence of the Acquired Immunodeficiency Syndrome," *Annals of Internal Medicine* 103 (1985): 670.

45. Heckler, "The Challenge," p. 656.

46. George Williams, T. B. Stretton, and J. C. Leonard, "AIDS in 1959" (letter), *Lancet* 2 (1983): 1126.

47. See Gina Kolata, "Boy's 1969 Death Suggests AIDS Invaded U.S. Several Times," *New York Times,* October 28, 1987.

48. Jay A. Levy et al., "Infection by the Retrovirus Associated with the Acquired Immunodeficiency Syndrome," *Annals of Internal Medicine* 103 (1985): 698.

▲ **CHAPTER 8.** How Diseases Change Their Meanings

1.   For a much more complete discussion of these and other changes in the meaning of the term "consumption," see Lester S. King's *Medical Thinking: A Historical Preface* (Princeton: Princeton University Press, 1982), pp. 16–69.
2.   Knud Faber, *Nosography: The Evolution of Clinical Medicine in Modern Times,* 2nd ed. (New York: Paul B. Hoeber, 1930; reprint, New York: AMS Press, 1978), p. 37.
3.   Ibid., pp. 38–39.
4.   King, *Medical Thinking,* p. 19.
5.   Ibid.
6.   Ibid., p. 44.
7.   Ibid., p. 47.
8.   Faber, *Nosography,* p. 99.
9.   Ibid., p. 79.
10.   Ibid., p. 101. Different strains of the tubercle bacillus, however, may produce different forms of tuberculosis, including scrofula.
11.   George L. Engel, "A Unified Concept of Health and Disease," *Perspectives in Biology and Medicine* 3 (1960): 463; F. Kräupl Taylor, *The Concepts of Illness, Disease, and Morbus* (Cambridge: Cambridge University Press, 1979), pp. 88–89.
12.   Engel, "A Unified Concept," p. 463.
13.   See F. Dudley Hart, "Gout and Non-Gout through the Ages," *British Journal of Clinical Practice* 39 (1985): 91–92; Thierry Appelboom and J. Claude Bennett, "Gout of the Rich and Famous," *Journal of Rheumatology* 13 (1986): 618–621; John H. Talbott, "Gout Therapy throughout the Ages," *Medical Times* 109, supp. (1981): 2–8; Kevin J. Fraser, "Anglo-French Contributions to the Recognition of Rheumatoid Arthritis," *Annals of the Rheumatic Diseases* 41 (1982): 335–343; James B. Wyngaarden and William N. Kelley, *Gout and Hyperuricemia* (New York: Grune & Stratton, 1976); and James B. Wyngaarden, "Gout," in *Cecil Textbook of Medicine,* 16th ed., ed. James B. Wyngaarden and Lloyd H. Smith, Jr. (Philadelphia: W. B. Saunders, 1982), pp. 1107–1118. For an alternative explanation of goutlike symptoms, see Richard Wedeen, *Poison in the Pot* (Carbondale: Southern Illinois University Press, 1984).
14.   For a more detailed description of typhoid fever, see Sherwood L. Gorbach, "Typhoid Fever," in *Cecil Textbook of Medicine,* 17th ed., ed. James B. Wyngaarden and Lloyd H. Smith, Jr. (Philadelphia: W. B. Saunders, 1985), vol. 2, pp. 1587–1589. For a historical discussion, see Harry F. Dowling, *Fighting Infection* (Cambridge: Harvard University Press, 1977), pp. 11–12, and John B. Thomison, "Typhoid Fever in Medical History," *Journal of the Tennessee Medical Association,* pt. 1, 67 (1974): 991–997; pt. 2, 68 (1975): 106–111; pt. 3, 68 (1975): 373–377.

15.   William Cullen, *First Lines of the Practice of Medicine, Including the Definitions of the Nosology,* ed. Peter Reid (Edinburgh: Bell et al., 1816), para. 32; Dale C. Smith, "The Rise and Fall of Typhomalarial Fever: I. Origins," *Journal of the History of Medicine* 37 (1982): 182–220; Lester S. King, *Transformations in American Medicine: From Benjamin Rush to William Osler* (Baltimore: Johns Hopkins University Press, 1990), pp. 47, 86–92, 93–116.

16.   Nathan Smith, *A Practical Essay on Typhous Fever* (New York: Bliss & White, 1821), reprinted in *Medical Classics* 1 (1937): 781–819; John Armstrong, *Practical Illustrations of Typhus Fever, of the Common Continued Fever, and of Inflammatory Diseases,* 1st American ed., from 3rd British ed., notes by Nathaniel Potter (Philadelphia: James Webster, 1821) and 2nd American ed., with corrections and appendix (1822), p. 14; Pierre Fidèle Bretonneau, *Traités de la dothinentérie et de la spécificité* (Paris: Vigot Freres, 1922; orig. published 1826); King, *Transformations,* pp. 72–79.

17.   W. W. Gerhard, "Reports of Cases Treated in the Medical Wards of the Pennsylvania Hospital, Part First," *American Journal of Medical Science* 15 (1834): 320–341; id., "Reports of Cases Treated in the Medical Wards of the Pennsylvania Hospital, Part Second," *American Journal of Medical Science* 16 (1835): 35–57; id., "On the Typhus Fever, Which Occurred at Philadelphia in the Spring and Summer of 1836; Illustrated by Clinical Observations at the Philadelphia Hospital; Showing the Distinction between This Form of Disease and Dothinenteritis or the Typhoid Fever with Ulceration of the Follicles of the Small Intestine," *American Journal of Medical Science* 19 (1837): 289–322; id., "On the Typhous Fever Which Occurred at Philadelphia in the Spring and Summer of 1836, Part Second," *American Journal of Medical Science* 20 (1837): 289–322; King, *Transformations,* pp. 86–92, 93–116; Robert Hudson, *Disease and Its Control* (New York: Praeger, 1987), p. 239; Esmond R. Long, *A History of American Pathology* (Springfield, Ill.: Charles C Thomas, 1962), p. 61; Leonard C. Wilson, "Fever and Science in Early 19th Century Medicine," *Journal of the History of Medicine* 33 (1978): 386–407; Dale C. Smith, "Gerhard's Distinction between Typhoid and Typhus and Its Reception in America, 1833–1860," *Bulletin of the History of Medicine* 54 (1980): 368–385.

18.   Elisha Bartlett, *The History, Diagnosis, and Treatment of Fevers of the United States,* 2nd ed. (Philadelphia: Lea & Blanchard, 1847); Austin Flint, "An Account of an Epidemic Fever Which Occurred at North Boston, Erie County, during the Months of October and November, 1843," *American Journal of Medical Science,* n.s., 10 (1845): 21–35; Austin Flint, *Clinical Reports of Continued Fever* (Buffalo, N.Y.: Geo. H. Derby, 1852), pp. 242, 246–247; Joseph M. Smith, "Report of the Committee on Practical Medicine," *Transactions of the American Medical Association* 1 (1848): 118, 120–122, 130; Henry F. Campbell, "An Inquiry

into the Nature of Typhoidal Fever; Being a Consideration of Their Theory and Pathology," *Transactions of the American Medical Association* 6 (1853): 453, 454, 461, 470–471.

19. Rufus Cole and Henry T. Chickering, "Typhoid Fever," in *A Handbook of Practical Treatment,* ed. John H. Musser and Thomas C. Kelly (Philadelphia: W. B. Saunders, 1917), vol. 4, p. 183; Charles-Edward Amory Winslow, *The Conquest of Epidemic Disease* (Madison: University of Wisconsin Press, 1971), p. 79; H. Gradle, *Bacteria and the Germ Theory of Disease* (Chicago: W. T. Keener, 1883); George Sternberg, *A Manual of Bacteriology* (New York: William Wood & Co., 1893), p. 216; William Osler, *The Principles and Practice of Medicine,* 2nd and 6th eds. (New York: D. Appleton & Co., 1896 and 1905).

20. Julia Older, *Endometriosis* (New York: Charles Scribner's Sons, 1978), p. 15.

21. James W. Curran, "The Epidemiology and Prevention of the Acquired Immunodeficiency Syndrome," *Annals of Internal Medicine* 103 (1985): 657.

22. Ibid.; "Proposed New Definition of AIDS Could Boost Cases 20%, Scientist Says," *Boston Globe,* March 18, 1987. The definition of AIDS could change again if recent discoveries of a second virus pan out. In 1987, French doctors discovered that certain patients showing symptoms of AIDS or ARC had a virus in their blood different from the HIV-1. This second virus, called HIV-2, resembles the HIV-1 but has some distinct genes. Thus, two different viruses appear to cause the "same" disease. We may ultimately view these differently caused conditions as different diseases, or we may continue to view them all as one disease (just as we do today with colds, something we consider to be one disease but which is actually caused by many different viruses). See "AIDS-Related Virus Raises Fears of New Epidemic," *Boston Globe,* May 7, 1987. Similarly, preliminary observations suggest that women infected with HIV may show clinical manifestations that differ from those included in the current case definition; these data could cause the numbers of people with "AIDS" to increase again. As of June 1991, however, the Centers for Disease Control report that, although studies are under way to clarify the natural history of HIV infection in women, "currently there is no scientific evidence that conclusively links HIV infection to life-threatening illnesses specific only to women."

23. Some might also argue that the meaning of "AIDS" changed once again in 1989, when many researchers were suggesting that merely carrying the virus would lead inevitably to death. If we may ignore the fallacies inherent in the notion of "inevitable" death from *any* disease, such a change in meaning would simply illustrate a sound principle: ailments may change their natures through political-scientific decisions, but each individual continues to have his or her unique and unchanged complaint and ultimate outcome.

24. See, for example, "What's News—World Wide," *Wall Street Journal,* No-

vember 2, 1990, and David Gelman, "The Brain Killer," *Newsweek,* December 18, 1989, pp. 54–56.

25.   See L. J. Rather, *Genesis of Cancer* (Baltimore: Johns Hopkins University Press, 1978), for a historical overview of the meaning of "cancer." Until improved microscopy allowed the development of tissue theory and, later, cell theory, scientists had limited tools with which to distinguish one mass from another (pp. 4–10).

26.   John C. Gunn, *Gunn's Domestic Medicine,* a facsimile of the 1st edition, with an introduction by Charles E. Rosenberg (Knoxville: University of Tennessee Press, Tennesseana Editions, 1986), pp. 284–285; originally *Gunn's Domestic Medicine; or, Poor Man's Friend* (Knoxville: "Printed under the immediate superintendence of the author, a physician of Knoxville," 1830).

27.   For a complete list of rheumatic diseases, see table 103–1 in *The Merck Manual of Diagnosis and Therapy,* 14th ed., ed. Robert Berkow (Rahway, N.J.: Merck, Sharp & Dohme Research Laboratories, 1982), pp. 1168–1171. This table is a modified version of the American Rheumatism Association's classification, "Primer on the Rheumatic Diseases," *JAMA* 224 (1973): 678–679.

28.   For an excellent discussion of this problem, see Ray Fitzpatrick, "Lay Concepts of Illness," in *The Experience of Illness,* ed. Ray Fitzpatrick et al. (New York: Tavistock Publications, 1984), pp. 11–31.

29.   D. W. Blumhagen, "Hypertension: A Folk Illness with a Medical Name," *Culture, Medicine, and Psychiatry* 4 (1980): 197–227.

30.   See I. N. Stevenson, "Editorial Comment," *Social Science and Medicine* 14B (1980): 1, for a discussion of this unconscious translation.

31.   James Alexander Hamilton, "The Identity of Postpartum Psychosis," in *Motherhood and Mental Illness,* ed. I. F. Brockington and R. Kumar (New York: Grune & Stratton, 1982), pp. 13–14. In this same book, G. Stein makes the same point, noting that "depression" is used to denote a symptom (Stein, "The Maternity Blues," p. 129).

32.   James Alexander Hamilton (personal communication).

33.   For example, see F. H. Spracklen, "The Chronic Fatigue Syndrome (Myalgic Encephalomyelitis)—Myth or Mystery?" *South African Medical Journal* 74 (1988): 448–452; Jane Dawson, "Royal Free Disease: Perplexity Continues," *British Medical Journal* 294 (1987): 327–328; E. Byrne, "Idiopathic Chronic Fatigue and Myalgia Syndrome (Myalgic Encephalomyelitis): Some Thoughts on Nomenclature and Aetiology," *Medical Journal of Australia* 148 (1988): 80–82; L. Renfro et al., "Yeast Connection among 100 Patients with Chronic Fatigue," *American Journal of Medicine* 86 (1989): 165–168; P. Manu, T. J. Lane, and D. A. Matthews, "The Frequency of the Chronic Fatigue Syndrome in Patients with Symptoms of Persistent Fatigue," *Annals of Internal Medicine* 109 (1988): 997; G. P. Holmes, "Chronic Fatigue Syndrome: A Working Case Definition," *Annals of Internal Medicine* 108 (1988): 387–389; P. Manu,

D. A. Matthews, and T. J. Lane, "The Mental Health of Patients with a Chief Complaint of Chronic Fatigue: A Prospective Evaluation and Follow-up," *Archives of Internal Medicine* 148 (1988): 2213–2217; A. S. David, W. Wessely, and A. J. Pelosi, "Postviral Fatigue Syndrome: Time for a New Approach," *British Medical Journal* 296 (1988): 696–699; M. J. Kruesi, J. Dale, and S. E. Straus, "Psychiatric Diagnoses in Patients Who Have Chronic Fatigue Syndrome," *Journal of Clinical Psychiatry* 50 (1989): 53–56; E. J. Bell, R. A. McCartney, and M. H. Riding, "Coxsackie B Viruses and Myalgic Encephalomyelitis," *Journal of the Royal Society of Medicine* 81 (1988): 329–331; L. C. Archard et al., "Postviral Fatigue Syndrome: Persistence of Enterovirus RNA in Muscle and Elevated Creatine Kinase," *Journal of the Royal Society of Medicine* 81 (1988): 326–329; K. Kroenke et al., "Chronic Fatigue in Primary Care: Prevalence, Patient Characteristics, and Outcome," *JAMA* 260 (1988): 929–934; D. Buchwald, J. L. Sullivan, and A. L. Komaroff, "Frequency of 'Chronic Active Epstein-Barr Virus Infection' in a General Medical Practice," *JAMA* 257 (1987): 2303–2307; E. J. Jacobson, "Chronic Mononucleosis—It Almost Never Happens," *Postgraduate Medicine* 83 (1988): 61–65; P. O. Behan and W. M. Behan, "Postviral Fatigue Syndrome," *Critical Reviews of Neurobiology* 4 (1988): 157–178; Ron Winslow, "CDC to Study Illness Derided as 'Yuppie Flu,'" *Wall Street Journal,* November 19, 1990; A. L. Komaroff, "Chronic Fatigue Syndromes: Relationship to Chronic Viral Infections," *Journal of Virology Methods* 21 (1988): 3–10; F. G. Jennekens and J. van Gijn, "Postviral Fatigue Syndrome or Myalgic Encephalomyelitis," *Nederlands Tijdschrift Geneeskunde* 132 (1988): 999–1001; "Chronic Fatigue: All in the Mind?" *Consumer Reports,* October 1990, pp. 671–675; Geoffrey Cowley, "Chronic Fatigue Syndrome: A Modern Medical Mystery," *Newsweek,* November 12, 1990, pp. 62–70; and Gregg Charles Fisher, *Chronic Fatigue Syndrome: A Victim's Guide to Understanding and Coping with This Debilitating Illness* (New York: Warner Books, 1989).

34. The same might be said in regard to neurasthenia and the chronic pain syndrome associated with depression or anxiety. The former disease hasn't been commonly diagnosed in the United States since early in the twentieth century, but it is widespread among psychiatric patients in the People's Republic of China. The same patients diagnosed as having "neurasthenia" in China could well be diagnosed as having "chronic pain syndrome" in the United States. See Arthur Kleinman, *Social Origins of Distress and Disease: Depression, Neurasthenia, and Pain in Modern China* (New Haven: Yale University Press, 1986), p. 79.

35. Rachmiel Levine, "History of Etiology of Diabetes Mellitus," *Archives of Pathology* 78 (1964): 405–408; Morris Notelovitz, "Milestones in the History of Diabetes—A Brief Survey," *South African Medical Journal* 44 (1970): 1158–1161; Frank N. Allan, "Diabetes before and after Insulin," *Medical History* 16 (1972): 266–273; Folke Henschen, "On the Term

Diabetes in the Works of Aretaeus and Galen," *Medical History* 13 (1969): 190–192; Leonard Mastbaum, "Diabetes Mellitus: Past, Present, and Future," *Minnesota Medicine* 62 (1979): 9–11; Chalmers L. Gemmill, "The Greek Concept of Diabetes," *Bulletin of the New York Academy of Medicine* 48 (1972): 1033–1036; T. Schneider, "Diabetes through the Ages: A Salute to Insulin," *South African Medical Journal* 46 (1972): 1394–1400; "Sugar in the Blood and Urine of Diabetic Patients," *American Journal of Medical Science* 26 (1840): 240; Terra Ziporyn, "Abnormal Insulin Molecules: An Alternative Cause of Diabetes?" *JAMA* 252 (1984): 2669–2670, 2673.

36. Similarly, some doctors argue that fibrocystic breast disease should be considered a nondisease as well, since the term has lost its specificity and refers to many different conditions. See Susan M. Love, Rebecca Sue Gelman, and William Silen, "Fibrocystic 'Disease' of the Breast—a Nondisease?" *New England Journal of Medicine* 307 (1982): 1010–1014.

▲ **Conclusion.** The Courage to Admit Ignorance

1. For detailed discussions of practical coping strategies, see Linda Hanner, *When You're Sick and Don't Know Why: Coping with Your Undiagnosed Illness* (Minneapolis: DCI Publishing, 1991), and Michael Castleman's "Are You a Medical Mystery?" *Reader's Digest,* June 1991, pp. 185–192.
2. For example, see Howard Spiro, *Doctors, Patients & Placebos* (New Haven: Yale University Press, 1986).
3. George Bernard Shaw, *Three Plays* (New York: New American Library, 1985), pp. 268–269.

Index